R

CURRENT DILEMMAS IN MEDICAL-CARE RATIONING

A Pragmatic Approach

Henry A. Shenkin

University Press of America, Inc.
Lanham • New York • London

996 by
.merica,® Inc.
4720 Boston Way
Lanham, Maryland 20706

3 Henrietta Street
London, WC2E 8LU England

ISBN 0-7618-0238-X (cloth: alk: ppr.)

⊖™The paper used in this publication meets the minimum
requirements of American National Standard for information
Sciences—Permanence of Paper for Printed Library Materials,
ANSI Z39.48—1984

Contents

Introduction

Accessibility to medical care throughout the world has always been limited by the ability to pay for it, just as all other consumer items and services. Until well into the twentieth century this made little difference, because therapeutics had little, and often even a deleterious, influence on the course of disease. The fact that medical care was scientifically ineffective until relatively recently accounts, perhaps, for suggestions that its rationing now be defined differently from the dictionary definition of rationing in general. The dictionary definition of rationing is: "the allocation of a resource the supply of which is limited."[1] Mulloy proposes that, logically, medical-care rationing should be defined as: the constraint on consumption so that a "patient does not receive all the care that ... would be of benefit"[2]. Some also believe the term rationing when applied to medical care includes the notion of meting it out "according to principles of justice and efficiency."[3] Others choose not to view marketplace limitation of access to medical care as rationing, reserving that term only for the withholding of medical care from people who are willing and able to pay for it[4].

The mention of rationing to contain the costs of medical care as an alternative to the marketplace is politically unattractive. That is because the term rationing connotes the withholding of a commodity from, or limiting its supply for, some individuals. Thus other terms, such as "resource or asset allocations" or "priority settings" are often used instead. Nevertheless, to set priorities for consumer commodities, or allocate resources among them, also implies limitation on the supply of some consumer products in favor of others. A limit on resources allocated to medical care, sooner or later, leads to a denying of some of its services. Thus the terms "priority setting" and "resource allocation", when applied to medical care, are euphemisms for rationing.

Currently, the recent extraordinary worldwide acceleration in the cost of medical care, because of continual innovations and aging of populations, has initiated expanded discussion of the rationing of medical care. Despite this recent heightened interest in medical-care rationing, and despite its always having existed everywhere, there is no comprehensive account of its various parameters. Rather, books on rationing tend to concentrate on one or another of its aspects, like ethical considerations[5], or how rationing should be applied to some particular therapeutic modalities[6], or on the problems in creating priorities for the rationing of medical care[7,8,9].

The purpose of this survey, then, is to collate the various parameters of medical-care rationing -- the reasons for it, the available methods for rationing, an examination of the philosophical principles that have been, and could be, used to determine how it is to be done, and finally its political realities in a democracy. In particular, it is intended to enlarge the approach generally applied to problems of medical-care rationing from one based only, all too often, on deductive reasoning and also consider the application of inductive reasoning to such problems. That is, to proceed from observed facts to general conclusions instead of only considering solutions based on *a priori* presumptions of what are the correct foundation for medical-care rationing and the proper methods for its operation. It is intended to suggest, for the readers' consideration, directions that possibly might be pursued in seeking answers to such problems - answers that are derived from observations of human nature and its effects on the development of democratic societies and their cultures.

Acknowledgements: I would like to thank David Smith, Ph.D., Budd N. Shenkin, M.D., MAPA, Reva Stein Kaplan, B.A., M.F.A., and Jane Tompkins, Ph.D. for their help and useful comments in the preparation of this book.

Chapter 1

Why of All Consumer Items Should Medical Care Be Rationed Other Than By the Marketplace ?

In recent years, observers in all nations have assumed, even if only tacitly, that it is medical care of almost all products and services which needs to be rationed by means other than, or in addition to, the marketplace. The outstanding explanation for this assumption has been the recent sky-rocketing costs of medical care - in a large part due to the introduction of insurance for medical care, which tended to counteract its rationing-by-the-marketplace. Then, the transfer of the costs of paying the premiums for insurance from individuals to their employers or to the state added to the costs of doing business and increased taxation. This now has become alarming to companies and to voters.

All advanced nations have seen fit to transfer resources from the more affluent to the less affluent. This has occurred because western mores dictate, and the public supports, that there be such a transfer of resources to make it easier for the poor and the weak to obtain all consumer items necessary for a minimal standard-of-living. Indeed, this applies especially to medical care because of the perception, by the beginning of the twentieth century, that medical care was a necessity and, therefore, was to be included in the rights of any individual, and it was not to be limited by an inability to pay for it. This moral decision led to economic support for medical care being spread among a broader population through insurance schemes and, eventually, direct governmental support. This development markedly increased the demand for medical services, not only because it made it available to more people but also because it caused medical services to appear to be of no cost to the individual at the time of its use. Later, when it became customary for employers to pay the insurance premiums of their employees, a practice subsidized by governments by making such contributions tax-exempt, it further distanced the individual from the costs of medical care.

More than 100 years ago, western European organizations created insurance societies to lighten the costs of illnesses for the individual since insurance makes the costs of medical care less onerous to any one individual by spreading the costs among many. Those insurance schemes (called sickness funds) at first were available only to the employed. Later, insurance plans were extended ever more widely. Most plans transferred wealth from the younger and healthier portion of the population to the older and sicker portion - whose care costs far more - by charging everyone the same premium ("community-rated" premium). Western European governments eventually paid the premiums for the poor and unemployed until essentially universal coverage had been achieved. In paying these insurance premiums for the poor, government is still transferring resources from the more affluent to the less affluent, but by means of its taxing power.

In the mid-twentieth century, the governments of Scandinavia, Britain and Canada guaranteed universal coverage almost entirely through taxation. At the same time, private medical insurance schemes became available in the U.S. Eventually, the government subsidized such plans by making the cost of premiums tax deductible for businesses, and exempting workers from having to declare these premiums as income. The rise of insurance schemes in the U.S. was followed, in 1965, by Medicare and Medicaid legislation to insure access for the elderly and the poor, respectively. Nevertheless, by the early 1990's, 16 to 17% of the U.S. population were still uninsured.

The methods utilized for broadening access to medical care have been called "zero-priced" ones, meaning medical care is made free to patients, or at least appears to be free when used. Such systems enhance the desire of individuals for medical care which, as is well-known, can be insatiable under such a circumstance[10]. Therefore, any zero-priced entry system, without rationing, can soon become unaffordable even to the wealthiest of nations (such as the U.S.) long before universal access is attained[11,12]. In addition, remuneration to providers in the U.S. has been uncontrolled. Providers, indeed, have had an incentive to increase their services, because "the more they did, the more they made."

Medical-care enfranchisements, in addition to increasing access and use, also increase costs by widening expectations of the breadth and amount of medical services available. For instance, even of those Americans insured, as many as 21% (@42,000,000) believe the benefits of their insurance plans are insufficient. Many people complain about insufficient and limited coverage, and lack of catastrophic and long-term provisions[13].

It is well recognized that increasing access to medical care without apparent cost to the individual so distorts the market that it no longer can control prices nor contain expenditures. The marketplace, anyway, tends to fail to adequately control medical-care prices because, even if individuals have to pay out-of-pocket for each item, medical care is so intricate and health concerns so often emotionally crushing, they cannot be knowledgeable purchasers, as is required for a market to control costs.

The transfer of the costs of medical care from the individual to the community not only removed the restraint of marketplace rationing on individuals but also creates a dilemma for the proponents of patient-autonomy as the keystone for medical ethics, and for rationing only explicitly (see Chapter 3, below). Such a dilemma arises when patients insist on treatments that well could benefit them but are not cost-effective (see page 32), or when families insist on prolonging the life of non-sentient individuals at great public expense[14].

When a goodly part of medical-care costs were transferred from the private to the public sphere, medical care had to compete with other services for public funds. This served as another factor leading to the perception of the need to ration medical care by means other than the marketplace. This facet of socialism, transferring resources from the more affluent to the less affluent, is still popular in capitalist economies despite the recent collapse of the socialist economies of eastern Europe, and despite economies more reliant upon the marketplace to set the amounts and prices of available items having proven to be more efficient in producing consumer items and raising a population's standard-of-living.

In addition to its morality, transferring the costs of medical care to governments is justified on the pragmatic basis that improving people's health helps them perform better in the workplace, thus benefiting the national economy[15]. This argument, however, runs up against studies indicating that equalizing therapeutic medical care is probably not economically cost-effective. Thus, contrary to our moral sense, some have suggested abandoning such efforts[16]. Observations that even equal access to care does not produce health equality within a nation's population[17,18,19] further support the argument against equalizing efforts. In addition, because socioeconomic factors govern many important causes of death more than does medical care[20,21], it has been suggested that the single most effective way to improve a nation's health would be to redistribute all resources more equally, not just medical care[16,22,23].

Other important factors leading to calls for the rationing of medical care have been the sharp accelerations in its costs occasioned by the remarkable technological innovations in therapeutic care and the aging of the population in recent decades. Even in the most advanced industrial nations these increasing costs are said to outstrip their ability to pay for medical care[6,24]. Indeed, it is medical care for the elderly and disabled portions of populations that are most often directly subsidized by governments, and the expansion of these portions of the population are due, in no small measure, to advances in health care over the last 100 years.

Also, since medical care is labor intensive, its share of the GNP of an expanding nation would have to constantly grow in comparison with other industries that are not labor intensive - such as those that make cars and computers. Therefore, one way to maintain parity among various items in an expanding nation's GNP is to hold the costs of medical care in check by rationing it more intensively[25].

Still another economic argument for rationing medical care by means other than by the marketplace is that the savings occurring from its capital-intensive innovations are never passed on to consumers, not even after recovery of the original investment. The same causes already mentioned (zero-priced methods, patients' ignorance of the product, etc.) that distort the medical-care market in general, also prevent passing on savings from medical innovations to the consumer. Furthermore, even when an innovation is more cost-effective than the treatment it replaces, it still tends to add to medical care costs. Such innovations, since they generally simplify treatment or treat a previously untreatable condition, often are used more frequently. For instance, laparoscopic cholecystectomy, introduced in 1988, is far less expensive than open, or surgical, removal of the gall bladder. However, by 1993 many more gall bladders were removed by laparoscopy than had been removed by open surgery in 1988, so that the total costs for gall bladder removal increased despite the decline in unit cost. The increase in gall bladder removals by laparoscopy occurred because it is a less risky procedure than open cholecystectomy and therefore available to an increased number of patients, including older ones.

Finally, is it possible that policy experts choose medical care, despite its present importance to well-being and longevity, for non-marketplace rationing rather than other consumer goods or services because the innovations which led to the industrial revolution came on-line long before the scientific breakthroughs that have made medical care really effective[26]? Creations of machinery, uses of energy, improvements in transportation and the development of the many goods for human consumption dominate our economic thinking and are now considered to be the basis for expanding national economies. The shifting of our economic focus, after the industrial revolution and the maturation of capitalism, from production to consumption further fostered a cultural emphasis on immediate gratification, hedonistic pleasure, and short-term outlook. Production and use of consumer goods have become the lynch pin of many nations' economies[27]. This shift occurred long before innovations in therapeutics made medical care really effective.

Economists and politicians, to spur the economy, currently encourage consumer spending on items other than medical care[28]. Then, when the cost of providing universal medical care intrudes upon the nation's other resources and adds to national indebtedness, the problem is said to be the need to control the consumption of (i.e. ration) medical care. No one calls for controlling foreign travel, or limiting the number of cars, bathrooms or TVs people can acquire. While many policy makers say that the nations continued economic well-being depends on expansion of services, they apparently exclude medical services -- even though they will say that the point of economic activity is the contribution it makes to the well-being of a population[29]. While politicians continue to propose controlling medical expenditures that, on balance, could be harmful to the overall economy of the nation[30], many communities try to repair their local economic depression by building expensive convention centers and other facilities to attract tourism, or by legalizing casino gambling (which in the U.S. had tripled over the past 30 years and, by 1993, was more than a $30 billion industry[31]) - never by planning more and better labor-intensive medical-care facilities.

Before 1940, medical care had not yet begun its advanced innovative stage. Before then, although many factors resulting from an improving economy did extend life, medical care by way of therapeutics could do little to affect longevity or the quality-of-life. Thus expenditures on medical care were not perceived as necessary and important to the economic viability of the nation. In 1936, longevity in the U.S. averaged only 60 years[32]. Increased wealth, better nutrition, and public-health measures had extended longevity from 37 years in 1875.[25]. Up to about 1965, the treatment of illness did not drain any individual economically, let alone strain any nation's economy, and the rationing of medical care could never be in question. While the ability to pay did affect the medical attention a patient received, for the most part, the resulting lack of attention didn't matter to a patient's physical health. In fact, it was often the case the less medical care a patient received, the better - then the patient would escape popular but misguided treatments like bleeding, purging, tonsillectomy, uterine suspension or lobotomy. But then, since the 1950's, innovations in medical care increasingly have helped extend longevity (which averaged 76.7 years in the U.S. in 1993) and helped improve the quality-of-life[33,34] and, probably, now contributes to "demographic efficiency" with its consequent accumulation of wealth[29]. However, these innovations, which can prolong life and improve its quality, have been very costly. They, along with aging of the population and increased access, now constitute the principal causes of sky-rocketing medical-care costs. And these cost factors are posing a most intractable problem.

The origin of the idea that unlimited consumerism and development of services are essential for a nation's economic well-being rather than unlimited expenditures in a medical-care industry devoted to extending life and improving its quality could be the factor of chance in the evolution of culture (just as chance plays a part in biologic evolution). If circumstances had created the technology to extend meaningful life prior to, or even simultaneously with, the technology used to make consumer goods, a nation's economy might then have depended on the continuing expansion of healthcare employment and expenditures for life-preserving technology rather than, or as well as, on consumerism or expanding service industries.

If innovative development had had a different economic time table, would cultural evolution have caused our policy experts to encourage spending on medical care rather than on consumer goods? If so, then to avoid excessive debt, expenditures on other sectors of the economy would have had to be curtailed in order to keep the total of expenditures equal to a nation's GNP. That is not to imply that the present order of priorities is incorrect, because until very recently a nation's health was determined more by its economic success than by the amount it spent on medical care, and some say much is still the circumstance[35].

The suggestion that national spending priorities should always put health expenditures at the top of the list certainly is not now realistic, but priorities can change. Economists have recently come to realize the value of increased investment in preventive public health is not only to the well-being of a population but also as an aid to the accumulation of its wealth[29]. Conceivably, their future studies will reveal that increased investments in therapeutic medical care will help to increase wealth as well as well-being.

Since all advanced nations are experiencing constantly accelerating expenditures on medical care, they all are seeking to ration medical care by means other than by the marketplace. On the other hand, policy experts don't entirely agree on how best to allocate their nation's resources to attain the best health and well-being of their populations, since it is agreed that should be the objective of all societies. In particular, they cannot decide in what proportions resources should be allocated to economic growth and "social justice" or to medical care. Most social scientists clearly prefer dedicating resources to economic growth and narrowing the gap between the rich and the poor, and reducing resources for medical care even if such a reduction would lessen the amount of medical care now received by the poor[36].

Such an attitude is confirmed by data in a study cited in a recent report of the British Labor Party's Commission on Social Justice. That data revealed, that despite their universal access to medical care, the longevity of inner city residents of Sheffield and Glasgow averaged eight years shorter than the suburban residents of those cities[37]. While this is a vivid example of the effect of affluence on longevity in Britain, that effect could be even greater in the

U.S. where difference in affluence between social classes is even greater than in Britain and, in any event, the population is less homogeneous.

One social scientist, impressed by the British data revealing how much healthier the affluent are than the poor, believes "it makes economic and social sense to limit spending on health care to free resources for other policies that promote health. Investing in health remains a worthwhile objective, but it means much more than spending on the NHS."[38]   Again, while reducing the economic discrepancy between the rich and the poor might well improve the health of the latter, if that led to reducing governmental support for their National Health Service (NHS), it would also exacerbate the perceived necessity for the NHS to ration its reduced amount of medical care.

The belief that only socioeconomic factors are of importance to health, and denigrating the role of medical care, appears to color the attitude of social scientists in discussing any aspect of medical-care rationing. This position of social scientists may in great part result from their use of a nation's average longevity and average infant mortality as the criteria for comparing the relative health of nations. Average national longevity and average national infant mortality by themselves are inadequate for such a purpose, since they do not reflect the comparative well-being of the various classes in the populations[39].

For instance, the average longevity is less and infant mortality greater in the U.S., despite its far greater expenditures on therapeutic medical care, are inferior to such data in other advanced nations comprising the Organization for Economic Cooperation and Development (O.E.C.D.). The conclusion is then drawn that the amount spent on therapeutic medical care, above a certain limit, has little or no relationship to the health of a nation's population. However, it is not pointed out that: those other

O.E.C.D. nations have more homogeneous populations than does the U.S.; that there is a greater discrepancy in affluence between the social classes in the U.S.; that no one has evaluated the influence of the longevities and infant mortalities of the various social classes on the average longevity and infant mortality for a national population; nor are there data on each social class's utilization of, and expenditure on, medical care and their influences on each class's comparative well-being and longevity, and that all such information well could be buried in averages for an entire population. Moreover, the efficacy of therapeutic care is more clearly of importance to the well-being of a population than to its longevity, and well-being is a more difficult parameter to measure.

Nevertheless, national averages of longevity and infant mortality are used as evidence that social and economic equality are more important for health than simple access to medical care and as further justification to ration medical care rather than other national budget items. That evidence makes medical care by itself less important than other social entitlements in raising the level of national health. It is, therefore, less of a necessity[38].

However, other reports have found that clinical medical care does have a real effect on longevity and well-being of people[33,34], and few experienced practicing physicians doubt this to be true. A Milbank Quarterly Report recently estimated that if clinical services were provided more widely it would extend life expectancy of the entire populations of the U.S. and Britain an additional 1.5 to two years[34]. The report also stated that medical care can be credited with three of the roughly seven years of increased life expectancy in the U.S. and Britain since 1950.

When policy makers support limiting medical-care resources and, thus, rationing it, they accuse physicians with opposing views of being motivated only by their own economic interests[40,41]. But policy experts are not without prejudice against the medical profession. For example, they cite only treatments with questionable and unproven efficacies to support their position and extrapolate such unproven status to all of medical care. They ignore treatments and technological innovations of unquestioned benefit to well-being and longevity, innovations such as antibiotics and the many new other medications, cataract removal, joint and heart valve replacements, etc. Social and economic status are not unimportant determinants of health, but enthusiasm for those factors should not belittle the importance of modern therapeutic medical care to the health and well-being of the people to whom it is available.

In summary, the evolution of western culture has made access to medical care an individual right and notably reduced the role of the marketplace in controlling medical-care expenditures. Transferring payments for medical care from the private to the public sector had accentuated this process. Consequently, to control its explosive acceleration in costs due to this increased access and subsequent innovative advances and longevity, many people believe now, more than ever, it is required that the rationing of medical care be augmented (by means other than by the marketplace).

Chapter 2

What Parts of Medical Care Need to be Rationed ?

For policy-making purposes health care can be divided into two categories: public health care (or just health care) on the one hand and medical, or therapeutic, or clinical care on the other. Medical care consists of the diagnosis and treatment of diseases. Public health care encompasses problems affecting the health of the population as a whole, environmental health, and administration of health services. Public health also includes preventive care programs and attention to socioeconomic factors affecting people's health.

While all of preventive medicine can be considered to be in the category of "public health", the most important aspects of preventive care, because of their effectiveness for the health of an entire population, are such public health measures as cleansing of water supplies, improved nutrition, and immunizations. This was the preventive care responsible for the increase in longevity at the end of the 19th and the early part of the 20th centuries. Such preventive care measures are relatively inexpensive and, therefore, their rationing is unnecessary[23]. The crisis in health care costs now, at the end of the 20th century, is a result of the accelerating costs of therapeutic care. Those calling for non-marketplace rationing as a means to solving the current crisis in American health care are aiming only at therapeutic medical care.

Observers often confuse meanings of health care when comparing national medical-care delivery systems. Many of the statistics cited for comparison - average longevity, infant and maternal mortality, and incidence of low-birth-weight babies - are epidemiological data, which measure health crudely for an entire population, and depend principally on public-health measures and not on therapeutic, or medical care. Overall longevity and infant mortality are meaningful for measuring the effect of health care in backward nations but, to repeat, they do not adequately reflect the full impact of medical care on the longevity and quality-of-life of the numerous relatively affluent portions of the population in advanced industrialized nations.

While longevity statistics can reflect the efficacy of therapeutic care for the aged, and probably the state of their well-being, the full value of this relationship is obscured by using only average longevity and infant mortality as criteria for a nation's health and not subdividing the population according to its relative affluence and educational levels. That the average longevity is lower and the average infant mortality is higher in the U.S. than in other advanced nations, even though the U.S. is the most affluent and spends the most money on medical care, is used to disparage the very positive influence of medical care on the longevity and well-being of the many individuals who have as much of it as is needed[33,34]. Undoubtedly these very positive effects of medical care are obscured within the national averages for all social classes usually cited by some policy experts.

Despite the horror expressed at the huge expenditures on medical care in the U.S., the real costs of medical care from 1960 to 1990 also rose substantially in 15 of the 18

O.E.C.D. nations. In six of these countries, the acceleration in costs was greater than that in the U.S.[42] One reason for this accelerated rise in costs in O.E.C.D. countries is that medical care is labor-intensive. Such services cannot be automated or sped up, and thus made more productive. If doctors and nurses worked much faster than they do, the quality of their services would diminish. Therefore, efforts to curtail costs must either reduce services across the board, or ration them. However, it has been suggested that if reformers take the same route to hold down the runaway costs of education and law enforcement as they do for limiting the costs of medical care, future societies may well have luxuries beyond imagining, "but its people will be ignorant and violent."[42]

Averaged longevity and infant mortality statistics are used to rail against allocating resources for medical-care research in advocating the allocating of more resources to preventive care[43]. It is argued that increased preventive care, in addition, would be a cost-containing measure. This claim is made despite the report that poor health resulting from deprivation due to socioeconomic factors cannot be improved by measures that focus only on disease prevention[23] -- and despite the fact that preventive medicine is often more expensive than therapeutic care[44]. Redirecting efforts from innovative therapeutics to preventive medicine is particularly recommended as a cost-containing measure[45]. This "robbing Peter to pay Paul", especially without first relieving poverty might well not improve overall national health and even be counterproductive by depriving many of improved therapeutic care. An experienced observer believes   -that lessening support for innovative therapies "by financing preventive approaches with the resources needed to advance therapies" could be harming those with "diseases causing real pain and suffering."[46]

Calls for preventive care appeal to the prejudices of the public: one derived from the age-old adage that "an ounce of prevention is worth a pound of cure."; and another from the popular suspicion that doctors want people to get sick in order to increase their incomes. Thus preventive medicine campaigns gain momentum from the fact that the very words: "contain costs by preventing disease rather than getting and having the disease treated" are beguiling to almost everyone. Public spending for prenatal care presents a good example of apparently justified preventive spending because it avoids much of the high cost of complicated premature births and the care of low birth-weight infants. However, a closer look at relevant studies reveals that the cost-effectiveness of public spending on prenatal care is "more optimistic than scientific", and in fact is likely untrue, and "contributes to the medicalization of complex social problems."[47].

Preventive medicine, even by utilitarian reasoning, is a doubtful strategy for saving money. Screening large numbers of healthy people - many of whom may never develop a particular disease - to find the few who will, is not cost-effective[48]. Disease prevention measures and promotion of improved life-styles will likely make people live longer, but they then would develop even more expensive geriatric illnesses. Despite the realization that reducing health care costs for younger people in the work-place only defers costs to later for care for the aged (and shifts costs to Medicare from private insurance companies) a health project consortium strongly advocated a preventive care and public health campaign to reduce need for medical services[49]. On the other hand, "Maybe if you really want to cut services", one medical ethicist suggests, "you should make sure everybody drinks, smokes a lot, drives fast and carries a gun."[50] Nevertheless, during the recent medical-care reform debate, public-health officials insisted that preventive and public-health programs were not only beneficial to the health of the population but also would be cost-containment strategies[51]. That position, that preventive care is a cost-containment measure, had been put forth in support of the 1994 U.S. medical-care reform effort despite the clear evidence to the contrary having been reiterated in a review of the subject as recently as 1993[52].

One observer had reported that meta-analysis of multiple-risk-factor intervention trials showed no benefit[53]; and then a more recent multiple-risk-factor intervention study then showed that the intervention group actually fared much worse[54]. All of which led to the suggestion that: "General practitioners would do better to encourage people to live lives of modified hedonism, so that they may enjoy, in full, the only life that they are likely to have."[55]

An assessment of preventive home visits by public-health nurses in the Netherlands revealed that they had not been beneficial to the state of health of the general population of elderly people living at home, although they might be effective if restricted to subjects in ill health[56]. A study in Britain also predicted that the most cost-effective way to reduce the risk of coronary heart disease in general practice populations would be to target only high risk groups rather than universal screening and intervention methods[57]. However, an editorial in the British Medical Journal, after reviewing recent results of universal screening for the altering of life styles to prevent diseases, concluded that emphasis on prevention, by altering priorities, was severely interfering with "The key tasks of general practice ... helping patients to understand and cope with illness, relieving symptoms, and offering the occasional cure."[58]

It had been reported previously that harping on preventive medicine in order to improve the health of a nation distracts from the principal cause of the disparity in longevity and quality-of-life among different social classes[23]. According to those authors, there is a direct correlation between affluence on the one hand and longevity and its quality-of-life on the other. The explanation for this correlation did not lie in preventive health measures. Differences in life style imposed by social status could furnish an explanation. For instance, years ago, when smoking and a high fat diet were more prevalent among the wealthy, there was still a direct relationship between affluence and longevity[23]. Therefore, to improve public health, it is more effective to concentrate on repairing socioeconomic differences than on preventive medicine. That doesn't mean that most aspects of preventive medicine aren't of benefit to a population's health and well-being and worthy of support. It simply means that greater concentration on preventive medicine can't solve the problems of the costs and availability of medical care in the U.S. or elsewhere. Undoubtedly, some preventive care measures are good, and some can even be regarded as necessities, but clearly documented instances are indeed rare; and for the most part, many of the arguments for it are overstated, or even fatuous.

Medical, or therapeutic, care, needs to be separated into two categories when considering its rationing: necessary care, which prolongs life and improves its quality; and unnecessary care which does neither.

There can be no dispute about the desirability of eliminating unnecessary care to reduce the costs of medical care -- for example, the overuse of diagnostic studies and certain treatments, excessive administrative costs, and "defensive" medical practices. But eliminating all unnecessary care would lower costs to an acceptable level only temporarily, because the costs of necessary care (as defined above) would, nevertheless, continue to accelerate, albeit from a lower base. The ongoing aging of the population and ever more expensive innovations coming on-line (which, in turn, contribute to prolongation of aged life) would continue to accelerate costs. Sooner or later, therefore, a crisis in the costs of medical care would recur. Experience with the Medicare End-Stage Renal Disease Program in the U.S. over a period of 20 years demonstrates that escalation of medical care costs because of innovations cannot be prevented merely by eliminating the misuse or overuse of new forms of technology[59]. Therefore, when one speaks of rationing medical care, it is only necessary care that is the desirable resource which is in limited supply and in need of allocation by rationing[60,61].

Some observers, particularly scientists who seek to have medical-care reform include incentives to expand biomedical research, view medical-care innovations as a cost saving device[62]. They believe innovations not only improve the quality of care and save lives but also can reduce the cost of care. They claim that "skewed incentives in the current system have caused some innovations to be used in cost-increasing ways, leading some observers to believe, mistakenly, that medical innovations necessarily increase costs."

Money spent on better outcome studies and improved informational and record-keeping systems, theoretically, should be cost-effective. However, it is unclear that introducing new diagnostic tests and treatments decreases costs. There is some evidence that innovations often raise costs by increasing utilization, even if newer tests and treatments are cheaper per unit cost than the ones they replace (see laparoscopic surgery, page 9). In addition, savings from increased productivity of medical technology are not passed on to consumers in the distorted medical-care market, as they are in other markets for consumer goods. Finally, an innovation might not be cost-effective in some instances because the savings are calculated to arise from eliminating the cost of terminal care that patients would have needed had not the innovation been available to cure them. But such savings might be illusory, because they would only be the result of deferring the costs of the terminal care of younger individuals to a later time when the same individuals are older and then sure to suffer from geriatric diseases.

Some commentators -- notably supporters of a single-payer plan -- believe rationing of medical care in any form is unnecessary in the U.S., even with universal access to medical care. They believe improving the efficiency of the system and reducing administrative costs could avoid rationing, provided the same percentage of the U.S. GNP currently used for medical care is maintained. This percentage, however, is considerably larger than that expended by nations which now have single-payer plans[63]. One estimate of the administrative savings of switching the U.S. to a Canadian-like, single-payer system was $55 billion for the year 1991, sufficient to have provide the estimated $48.2 billion needed to cover the 35 million uninsured in the U.S. that year[63].

The supporters of a Canadian-like single-payer program for the U.S. imply that such a plan would prevent future acceleration of the proportion of the GNP spent on medical care, thereby permanently avoiding a cost-crisis. Reducing unnecessary care, including administrative costs, can undoubtedly diminish overall costs. Ultimately, however, after the initial savings from a single-payer plan are realized, some form of rationing would be necessary to counter the acceleration in expenditures on necessary care[61,64]. Rationing, after all, now takes place in Canada. This problem is often called the "residual argument": the rate of growth of medical care expenditures constitutes the real policy problem, not the absolute level of expenditures[65]. This explains why all advanced countries with aging populations, despite their varied levels of expenditure on medical care, and even those with single-payer systems, are experiencing, roughly, the same rates of acceleration in medical-care costs.

Fourteen percent of the growth in personal health care expenditures in the U.S. from 1960 to 1991 was due to medical care inflation beyond the general economy-wide inflation[66]. The reasons for this excess inflation in medical-care costs are the same as those presented above in section two that discusses why medical-care costs had been removed from the control usually exerted by a marketplace. Although eliminating sources of cost-escalation in medical care would be helpful, it would not offset the continuing rise in costs due to aging and technological innovations. Even if eliminating the inflation due to distortions of the medical-care marketplace could be achieved, it would not stave off the rationing of necessary care[67].

Another frequent suggestion for controlling medical-care costs and, by implication, avoiding rationing, is to enhance competition. There are two forms of suggested competition. The first, among providers, is called "managed competition"[68,69]. The second, among both insurers and providers, is labeled "competitive health markets"[70]. Both of these proposed suggestions for medical-care reform also encompass universal coverage and the provision of a guaranteed minimum health package, or plan.

Defining the contents of a health package clearly constitutes rationing, because it limits the less affluent to the medical care that is provided by any agreed upon minimum plan. Some argue that a minimum health plan would limit only unnecessary and useless medical care, and therefore does not connote rationing. Rudolf Klein, the English health-policy expert, counters, that "no country has yet designed such a package and it is difficult to see how it could be defined, given that changing technology is constantly redefining what medicine can do."[71]

In summary, only the therapeutic, or medical care, component of health care is expensive enough to require rationing. Even then, since "unnecessary" medical care has no useful purpose, well-conceived legislation or regulation should be able to control it - leaving only necessary medical care with the need to be rationed. Many observers have sponsored preventive care as the means to reduce the costs of "necessary" medical care and avoid its rationing. While most aspects of preventive care are important for better health, preventive care doesn't work for the purpose of saving money. The same statement holds for medical technology: it is important for good health, but very little of it can be looked upon as cost-saving. If costs of necessary care need to be curtailed, its rationing must be steadily intensified. Otherwise, the demand and costs for necessary care, care which either prolongs life or improves its quality, are sure to escalate constantly.

Chapter 3

How Can Medical Care be Rationed ?

A. General Categorization of Methods

As in economics, there are both "macro" and "micro" varieties of rationing. *Macro-rationing* occurs when governments limit the funds allocated to medical care, as by global budgeting or by establishing a single-payer mechanism that negotiates budgets with providers.

Global budgeting and single-payer plans permit a government or association of insurers to negotiate with all providers at one time and contain costs by reducing their profits and forcing them to be more efficient. For instance, hospitals can be led to agree to regionalization of facilities rather than competing with each other to acquire them, the latter practice most often leading to under-utilization or unnecessary utilization.

Macro-rationing decisions such as global budgeting -- often sooner rather than later -- lead to deciding which individual can have specific procedures whose supply is limited by the total of funds budgeted for medical care. Such decisions, at the level of the individual patient, would be examples of *micro-rationing*.

Another useful classification for the understanding of the functioning of rationing methods is dividing them by whether they are explicit or implicit. ***Explicit rationing*** occurs when rationing is done openly by law or governmental regulation and rules and, therefore, is "visible" to the public. ***Implicit rationing*** occurs when decisions about who receives medical care and what sort are not legally mandated but are made by the nature of the delivery system.

All macro-rationing decisions are, by definition, more or less explicit. For instance, in Great Britain, as part of the 1991 reforms of the NHS aimed at creating an internal market, health authorities and health boards were told to assess the needs of the populations they serve in order to set priorities in allocations of their portion of the Government's budget for medical care. This is a difficult goal to achieve. Britain is now using a system of "weighted capitation allocations" in an effort to assure equitable distribution of the globally budgeted funds among the various regions[72]. Weighted capitation provides a formula for adjusting population projections to take account of each region's needs and the costs of providing medical care. Needs are adjusted by national variations in the use of hospital beds by different age groups, and by a measure of standardized mortality associated with regional variations in hospital use.

However, as definitive as weighted capitation sounds, NHS policy makers felt that equalizing allocations still called for more and improved research[73]. They were led to this conclusion, for instance, because allocating assets according to prior costs penalizes England's inland regions, since many older people had retired from those regions and moved to the seashore. This migration of the elderly has markedly increased medical-care costs in seashore regions and inflated their allocations as compared with inland regions. This is viewed as an illegitimate distortion favoring care for the aged and reducing resources that could provide greater benefits for younger people[74].

A medical economist also criticizes the determination of priorities according to the total needs of a region because he believed it ignored costs and failed to take into account the potential benefits for patients from treatment or prevention[75]. This economist recommends instead using marginal analysis, i.e., beginning with the existing pattern of expenditure of resources and examining the effects of small changes to that pattern. "Marginal analysis focuses solely on the extra costs and benefits of changes in expenditure of resources. It analyses the effect of shifting resources between programmes - that is, changing the balance of expenditure. Overall efficiency will increase when the marginal gain in benefit in the expanding programme exceeds the marginal loss of benefit in the contracting programmes. As a result, marginal analysis identifies where additional resources should be targeted, where reductions should be made if expenditures must be cut, and how resources should be reallocated to achieve overall gain in benefit with no overall gain in expenditure."[75]

Other analysts believe that, even with more sensitive indicators of need, important policy questions would still remain unanswered[76]. Such questions include, for example, the following: should resources be redistributed to relatively deprived inner city areas at the expense of more affluent parts of the country? While British policy experts are gathering large amounts of data on epidemiologically-assessed healthcare needs[77], it is unclear whether the public will accept this approach to explicit rationing.

In Canada, public-health policy experts believe that, morally, public-health resources should be allocated according to the needs of the population, not according to the needs of health care facilities and providers[21]. However, it also has been noted that the health of individuals correlates most closely with their socioeconomic status, not with their accessibility to care. (This correlation occurs even where there is universal access and after controlling for age, race, gender, baseline health status, smoking, alcohol consumption and exercise.) Therefore, using the medical needs-of-the-population as the determining factor in allocating healthcare resources would have little effect on the general health of people. In view of this, and lack of availability of still other data for making allocations according to the needs-of-the-population, and the general requirement to minimize healthcare costs, the authors[21] recommended that expenditures should be equalized per capita, rather than according to facility usage. They also recommended that payment to providers should be determined not by fee-for-services but by the size and characteristics of the population served.

Where insurance plans for medical care have been introduced it needs to be remarked that just by setting the benefits covered they, in effect, ration medical care explicitly. As a matter of fact, in 1993 the prestigious Institute of Medicine debated what benefits should be included in the reform of the medical-care delivery system in the U.S.[78]. The Institute recognized that the current state-of-the-art research on cost-effectiveness and outcomes are clearly insufficient to set practice guidelines for settling what benefits should be covered. Their only conclusion was that health-plan coverage to be equitable should be flexible and people should trust the health-plan managers.

Even more recently, a frequent contributor to the literature on rationing suggests that explicit micro-rationing can be divided into two types: *rationing by exclusion* or *rationing by guidelines*[79]. With the former method, a list of conditions and their treatments are drawn up and ranked in order of their priority. Then, those conditions and their treatments are excluded from funding below a level of priority determined in consideration of the amount of resources available. This explicit method of micro-rationing has been carried out in Oregon for Medicaid with the objective of including as many eligible patients as possible in that program without increasing expenditures.

Guidelines for medical practice can be used for varying purposes depending upon how they are constructed. Their purpose could be exclusively to improve decision-making for the individual patient - if they be constructed solely as to effectiveness without consideration for their cost. By contrast, if an important factor in their construction be costs and the relation of the recommended decisions to budgets for medical care, then they should be considered as a method for micro-rationing. When practice guidelines are recommended to physicians practicing autonomously in their treatment of individual patients, they cannot be viewed as an explicit rationing procedure since the doctors would be free to use their professional ethics in accepting or rejecting a practice guideline[80]. On the other hand, when a physician's autonomy is limited by third-part payers or "managed care" organizations (see below, page 60) guidelines are a rationing mechanism since, then, cost considerations invariably participate in their formulation. These alternative purposes for practice guidelines once again reiterate the difference in attitudes that often exist between practicing physicians, with their professional ethics demanding their chief responsibility be to their individual patients, and policy makers who generally have the whole of society as their principal concern.

Explicit micro-rationing by guidelines is being done in New Zealand where a governmental committee drew up "guidelines for the treatment of specific conditions and the provision of different services. New Zealand's approach is based on the belief that priorities are best set by ensuring that patients who can clearly benefit from treatment receive access to care, rather than by excluding whole categories of services from public funding."[79] The author of this comment, a British policy expert, goes on to point out that, while Great Britain tends to micro-ration by guidelines, no one is willing to take the lead in furthering or enforcing such an unpopular issue as rationing. Consequently, he labels Britain's present method of keeping the NHS within its global budget as "rationing by muddling through".

Many people regard explicit micro-rationing as more just than implicit micro-rationing since it is implemented openly and applies equally to everyone. Such open implementation would presumably be less subject to manipulation. Indeed, most medical policy experts and social scientists prefer explicit rationing to implicit rationing by doctors[72,81,82].

Recently however, one frequently published expert gave many reasons to dissent from that prevailing attitude[83]. He points out that many in favor of explicit micro-rationing propose deriving the rules for it from quality-control and cost-effectiveness studies, but this, as will be elaborated upon below, is more easily said than done. Also, it is usually proposed to evaluate necessary healthcare modalities economically, a technique invented to assist in prioritizing a resource whose supply is limited[82]; but this technique is useful only for public sector investment planning where, unlike the private sector, individual costs, prices and profits are not available to guide investment decisions since goods and services are often provided free or, in the case of insured medical care, appear free at the time of consumption.

For economic evaluation of healthcare modalities, there are four main types: cost-minimization analysis, cost-effectiveness analysis, cost-utility analysis and cost-benefit analysis. All four types of economic analysis depend upon clinical evaluation of the effectiveness of the different treatments under consideration[84]. Unfortunately, such information is all too often unavailable[85]. Therefore non-empirical opinions or public desires frequently become the grounds for judgment. Evaluation of treatment outcomes is so difficult in fact, that one might wonder if valid judgment is ever possible, despite the optimism of those devoted to the subject[86].

Cost-minimization analysis is appropriate only when treatments are known to have the same outcome and the analysis is to identify the least cost option[87]. Cost-minimization can only be useful to conserve resources, not for rationing or prioritizing procedures.

Cost-effectiveness analysis, although often used loosely to refer to any economic evaluation, is a term appropriate only when evaluating procedures or programs with variable outcomes but whose comparative effectiveness can be expressed in a common natural unit[88]. For instance, one can evaluate treatments for hypertension by comparing the lowering of blood pressure in terms of millimeters of mercury. For treatment of other chronic diseases the unit of comparison can be the number of life-years gained. For diagnostic or screening procedures the comparative unit can be the number of positive cases detected and lives saved. Thus, cost-effectiveness analysis permits comparing procedures in terms of cost per unit. Cost-effectiveness studies can help conserve resources in the diagnosis and treatment of diseases by pinpointing the option providing the same result at the least cost. Cost-effectiveness studies, along with evidence of safety and efficacy, have been especially helpful in setting up guidelines for public reimbursement of the cost of drugs[89]. Cost-effectiveness is especially useful for eliminating medical services whose overall costs are so great in relation to the amount of benefit, or number of patients benefited, that a community cannot afford to supply them. However, it is difficult to establish just how many lives, or how much well-being, can be justifiably sacrificed and at what level of expenditure to define cost-effectiveness[90].

Some people even question whether it is ever ethical to sacrifice the well-being of any group, or even an individual, merely to save money. Certainly, the *rule-of-the-rescue* (*v.i.*) can make rationing decisions difficult to enforce. Despite the obvious attraction of cost-effectiveness studies, it has so far proven difficult to achieve cost-effectiveness data useful for the allocation of medical-care resources[46,72,78,91,92].

In evaluating the conflict between the individual and society created by cost-effectiveness studies, two leading analysts recommend that "physicians must broaden their perspective to balance the needs of individuals directly under their care with the overall needs of the population served by the health care system, whether the system is an HMO or the nation's health care system as a whole. Professional ethics will have to incorporate social accountability for resource use and population health as well as clinical responsibility for the care of individual patients."[44] This seems hardly more than a restatement of the problem and not really a solution. That is unless it is an advocacy to return to implicit rationing by physicians, a position opposed by most other policy experts and ethicists. Moreover, the more rationing is being openly discussed, "increasingly doctors seem unwilling to bear this responsibility on their own."[79]

Cost-utility analysis is used to compare treatments of different diseases or programs whose units of effectiveness vary. The outcomes of different procedures are measured in "utility" based units. Derived from the philosophical concept of utilitarianism, utility is a term economists use to express the subjective satisfaction that people derive from consuming goods or services[93]. In medical care, utility is the subjective level of well-being that people experience in different states of health. Setting priorities on this basis of individual preferences has been labeled a "bottom up" consultation, in contrast to "top down" decisions made by health authorities[94].

Some medical economists, to improve cost-utility analysis, have proposed using a measured quality-adjusted-life-year (QALY) to express the influence of interventions on the quantity and quality-of-life in terms of a single unit. They then compare costs per QALY gained[95]. QALY has been proposed to replace life expectancy as a more meaningful measure for outcomes even though it places greater demand on data and analysis. They have used various questionnaires to ascertain people's opinion of their state of health, and create standards from such data. The ultimate aim is to establish a QALY table to guide resource allocation decisions. Such a table would then help to shift resources from procedures costly in terms of the health benefits they generate, to those of relatively low cost[94].

Unfortunately, it is now known that patients' self-assessment of their life's quality under similar circumstances differ among themselves, as do their priorities[96]. Consequently, there is little agreement on the meaning of quality-of-life and so no unified approach has been developed to measure the quality-of-life[97]. Nonetheless, costed quality adjusted life-years have been used by the Oregon project to explicitly set priorities for allocating care to those poor people covered by Medicaid, so as to include many people previously uncovered without raising Medicaid costs inordinately[98,99].

Some have criticized the cost-utility analysis method of priority-setting: for discriminating against the elderly and the disabled (since the majority of respondents are young and able); for making illegitimate interpersonal comparisons; and for disregarding equity considerations[100,101]. Nevertheless, its proponents say that: "decisions have to be made about the allocation of resources and cost-utility analysis is probably the most sophisticated form of economic evaluation available at present."[93] Others have discarded measurement by QALY as likely to be subjective and potentially inaccurate[102,103].

Cost-benefit analysis can refer to any type of economic evaluation, but is usually restricted to analyses that place a monetary value both on costs and benefits of medical care. "... the attachment of monetary values ... makes it possible to say whether a particular procedure or programme offers an overall net gain to society in the sense that its total benefits exceed its total costs. Cost-effectiveness and cost-utility analysis do not do this because they measure costs and benefits in different units."[104]

There are several ways to put a monetary value on benefits. One method is to value medical services according to the wages earned when people return to work after a successful treatment. Another method is to establish how much people are willing to pay for a successful treatment. Either method enables comparison, in monetary terms, of returns on investment in medical-care procedures with any other kind of investment. However, some observers object that it is not valid to compare individual health and longevity with monetary returns from stocks or bonds.

Since quality-control and cost-effectiveness studies are almost completely unavailable[105,106], some policy experts hope to develop acceptable priorities through consultation with the public, even in the absence of a scientific basis for such a selection[105,107,108]. Such consultations seek to legitimize rationing by asking the people to identify what services they are most willing to forego, but the entire process has been labeled "The unaccountable in pursuit of the uninformed."[109]

For instance, public opinion surveys are remarkably sensitive to how questions are posed[110]. They inevitably discriminate against the healthcare needs of minority groups, especially by the young against the minority who are old[100,101], and certainly the perceived needs of the healthy differ from those of the unhealthy[111]. Polling the public on their perceived needs definitely does not promote equity[111]. Moreover, to legislate every nuance of care, and to whom and under what conditions it is to be supplied throughout a nation, is such a massive administrative job that there are sure to be many irrational decisions that will inflame the public and create massive dissatisfaction with the whole process of priority-setting. Varying patient preferences, as well as the difficulty in comparing procedures with different benefits for various patients, make it impossible to create rules - as for example, to explicitly ration surgical procedures[112].

Actually, surveys of the British public indicated it believes physicians can make the best decisions on rationing[7]. But then, efforts to openly impose guidelines on autonomous physicians' practices have so far proven to be fruitless. Studies of the efforts of the British NHS to mandate practice guidelines have shown that they are little likely to change behavior of doctors[113]. One experienced clinician-observer went even further, saying: "the idea that each element of medical practice will be dictated by systemic evidence-based research will be found to be as naive as the hopes of logical positivism that we can explain all of the universe, including ourselves, from Euclidian geometry."[114]

Finally, Rudolf Klein, Professor of Social Policy at the University of Bath, has concluded that: "there is no technological fix, scientific method, or method of philosophic inquiry for determining priorities. Of course, the three Es, - economists, ethicists, and epidemiologists - all have valuable insights to contribute to the debate about resource allocation and rationing, though none can resolve our dilemmas for us .... To put it another way, this is an argument that will never be finally settled,"[71].

While legislated explicit micro-rationing might seem fair in the abstract, when such laws (or directives) are actually applied those denied care and their families often will circumvent the directives by one means or another. This phenomenon is called the *rule-of-the-rescue*: no matter what the guidelines, individuals will obtain a treatment if it is known to exist. In addition, practitioners and policy experts will always disagree about treatments that are not cost-effective epidemiologically, yet can help individuals. The "rule-of-the-rescue" operates almost everywhere, and particularly among the more affluent and educated. Other analysts have suggested that the public's support, and desire, for constantly greater technological capability is an important underlying factor in the failure of managed-care organizations to more fully restrain medical-care costs[64]. Nor are physicians immune to the rule-of-the-rescue. Perhaps the most extreme illustration of this fact is neonatologists' insistence on expending huge sums on very premature infants who are bound to have many physical and cognitive impairments[115].

Some intensive-care physicians struggling to decide how to allocate their expensive facilities concluded that they must move away from patient's autonomy as the driving force in medical decision-making[116]. Such an opinion, of course, raises the ethical question of whether a physician must disclose to a patient all treatments available, or only those that can be afforded under the rationing directives in force[117]. In the U.S., intensive-care physicians say they are finding it difficult to recover the decision-making capacity from patients and relatives who traditionally "believe in the effectiveness of technology" and that "everything possible should be done for patients, without consideration of cost" and that "Both patients and health care providers believe in the 'rule-of-the-rescue'..."[116].

The rule-of-the-rescue is strengthened in the U.S. by the fact that anyone denied a treatment because of its costs can appeal to the courts. Courts then have to decide whether the treatment is medically necessary or appropriate to the individual plaintiff, regardless of any previous explicit rationing decision to forego such treatment[118]. Up to 1993, various U.S. courts had all decided in favor of the individual[119]. Later, the Americans with Disabilities Act of 1992 was extended to further contravene rationing decisions. That Act was used by a Federal Circuit Court as the basis for making a health insurer pay for even an unproven, experimental treatment[120]. The court was presumed to have based its opinion on the assumption that by failing to pay for the treatment, even if its efficacy was unproven, the insurer was discriminating against a woman disabled by breast cancer.

The perceived need to ration medical care is now so ubiquitous that two medical ethicists for instance, when discussing criteria for do-not-resuscitate (DNR) orders, felt compelled to remark that: " ..... disagreements over futility are actually debates over the prudent allocation of limited health care resources."[121] Indeed, this last statement again delineates the differing attitudes between medical policy experts and practitioners towards rationing in general. All rationing mechanisms imply the eventual denial of useful medical care to relatively few patients in favor of containing total costs of medical care for an entire society[122]. For instance, practitioners might believe that if there is one chance in five, or even in ten, that a patient would usefully survive a treatment then the situation is not futile and that treatment, no matter what the cost, should be allowed. Policy experts, on the other hand, in consideration of the economic cost involved in uselessly extending the life of four out of five patients, or more certainly regarding the saving of only one of nine of ten lives as not cost-effective, probably would regard the situation as futile and that treatment should not be provided[122]. Anyway, curtailment of presumed futile care has been found to save relatively little money[123,124]. Finally, complex statistical methods to predict futility for patients in intensive care units (ICUs)" are used to derive equations that fit observed mortality for populations but not for individual patients"[125]. These last authors go on to say that data from APACHE, MPM, SAPS, TISS and SUPPORT studies designed to predict when treatment of patients in ICUs is futile and a waste of resources "can provide support for experienced clinicians but must not be forged into weapons".

The severe expense of developing some foreseen new treatments, like gene therapy, no matter how well they serve individuals, benefit so few people that their cost-effectiveness ratios will be so skewed that they are sure to be assigned the lowest priorities. Therefore, those relatively few people benefited would be deprived by the current drive to contain costs through the rationing method that sets priorities through relative cost-effectiveness studies.

Some policy experts have suggested that no life-sustaining treatment be given after a certain agreed-upon age[126]. A related and appealingly rational-appearing suggestion is to abandon the great expenditures made during the last year of life as wasted efforts[127]. Singer and Lowry[127] also suggest that expanding the living-will initiative, by obtaining a patient's consent to withhold treatment in the last year of life, would ethically legitimatize such a practice. The problem with this proposal, however, is apparent to any practicing physician: how does one know when the last year of life begins? Anyway, the vast majority of physicians have always treated the terminal patient in accord with the usual directives suggested for the writing of a living-will. The available data, limited as they might be, confirm that any new proposals for saving costs at the end of life through the greater use of advance directives, DNR (do-not-resuscitate) orders, hospice care and by less aggressive interventions can only be the most modest[124,128]. Two experienced clinicians have observed: "Prediction models support decisions made by physicians, patients, families and third-party payers but they can be insensitive in respect of mortality" with regard to any individual.[125]

An ethicist contends that justice demands all treatments should be available to certain people, no matter how else they are rationed[129]. He argues that society has no right to remove all civil liberties, including the right to complete health care, from psychiatric or infectious patients confined against their will. "Even if specific rights to treatment cannot, for reasons of public financial prudence, be given to all NHS patients they must be given to psychiatric patients. Infringement of individual rights requires acceptance of social duties." A variation on this theme is the Americans with Disabilities Act of 1992 which gives disabled people special privilege by forcing their exemption to any rules for explicit rationing[130].

Explicit micro-rationing entails so many difficult procedural problems that it has not yet ever been utilized. Most people are not sufficiently altruistic to favor what is good for the greatest number that does not immediately benefit them, even if such a position could be better for themselves in the long run. Many people cannot defer present desires for future good and, in the case of illness, most people cannot willingly forego medical care for themselves or their kin[61,129]. Moreover, the public has far greater expectations than doctors or nurses of what medical care can accomplish, especially new technology, and are more demanding of it[23]. The biological evolutionary instinct for self-preservation drives people to act according to their own (immediately) perceived self-interest. This instinct can be one explanation for why explicit micro-rationing has never been implemented.

Nevertheless, increase in recent discussions of explicit rationing arise from the modern cultural trend to emphasize patient-autonomy and individual rights as the basis for medical ethics. Now that rationing of medical care is being more openly discussed, it will be interesting to see whether explicit rationing can be achieved in any society. All micro-rationing thus far has been implicit and, when not implemented by the marketplace, based on utilitarian principles. Rationing based on any other philosophy, such as Rawlsian justice (see page 70), would require explicit micro-rationing. Whether a democracy can carry out explicit rationing is by no means certain. Policy experts, non-etheless, frequently assume that public discussion can facilitate explicit rationing by helping people develop realistic expectations, by supplying informed consent to those to be deprived of some care, and by simultaneously providing "leadership resolve"[131].

Yet, can it ever be ethical to ration some treatments as, for example, to deny someone a known cure for a fatal disease because of the expense involved? For instance, it has been suggested that hospitals, to keep within a global budget, should sometimes deny patients curative drugs whose expense could be used for "better purpose" elsewhere[102]. Other such ethical dilemmas of the same nature arise when attempting to resolve certain unavoidable predicaments - - dividing a limited resource among an entire population and having to deny a resource to one group of people in order to make other resources available to a larger group.

Implicit rationing is usually micro-rationing implemented without open discussion, either according to the patient's ability to pay, or by physicians making case-by-case decisions. Physicians' implicit rationing decisions have been, and probably still are, most often made in the privacy of the home or their offices, and within the context of individual doctor-patient relationships. Physicians, when implicitly micro-rationing their care, consider the patient's age, likely prognosis and prospective quality-of-life. Implicit rationing by physicians is usually "invisible" to the general public. Political reality, so far, has dictated that, while many democratic nations have explicitly macro-rationed medical care - by single-payer plans, global budgeting and regionalization of facilities - micro-rationing has been carried out only implicitly in all nations.

All nations have widely employed implicit rationing. The way it operates in individual situations depends upon the individual's ability to pay for medical care or, particularly where there are global budgets, upon the beneficence of medical practitioners' judgments regarding not only the best interests of their patients but also the feasibility for society considering the circumstance in question and given the limitation on funds allocated to medical care[132].

The existence of many general practitioners with long-standing associations with their patients, along with respect for physicians built up over years of interpersonal relationships, are both necessary to make implicit micro-rationing by doctors possible. Free choice of doctors and continuity-of-care by one physician are also necessary for the adequacy of the doctor-patient relationship for this task. While there must be many exceptions, many observers believe that implicit rationing by physicians makes fair decisions more frequent than does reliance upon an across-the-board application of an ideal concept of justice[133,134].

Even in the U.S. where the marketplace often determines access, it is tacitly recognized that implicit rationing by physicians helps conserve resources[135]. Physicians, when rationing implicitly, base their decisions most frequently on the utilitarian principle of who would benefit the most from use of a limited resource comparing the conditions and ages of various patients. On the other hand, many observers believe that implicit rationing by doctors is an example of paternalism, and is not to be condoned[81].

To be effective and acceptable then, implicit micro-rationing requires a firm doctor-patient relationship with physicians practicing autonomously. In the U.S., the doctor-patient relationship has been seriously eroded for a variety of reasons. In the first place the American system makes specializing more attractive to medical students than general practice; the choice of general medical care is "low on their (students) own and their institutions priority lists."[136] There are now too few general practitioners with whom patients can establish a long standing relationship, and recognition of the greater educational requirements for specialists tends to denigrate GP's in the view of patients. Patients relationships to specialists, by definition, are limited. Moreover, specialists have a different view of their availability to patients than do general practitioners.

The inordinate increase in the affluence of doctors has been a second important factor in denigrating the respect for the medical profession. This increase in physicians' incomes followed upon the introduction of insurance systems which gave them recompense from many more patients on a fee-for-service basis while making medical care appear free to the patient at the time of use. Then again, previous to the scientific revolution in medical practice doctors were not held accountable for patients' undesirable responses to disease - as long as they were attentive. Now that advances have made medical care truly effective for many ills, people, under the emotional stress of sickness, have come to believe science can cure everything. Therefore, a poor outcome of treatment is no longer viewed as the result of unfortunate fate, but rather the physician's fault.

Finally, reducing the strength of the doctor-patient relationship is being abetted by many ethicists denigrating physician-beneficence in favor of patient-autonomy. One ethicist, for example, discussing patients' freedom to choose their own medical care, recently wrote: "It is not medicine's responsibility to prevent tragedies by denying freedom, for that would be a greater tragedy."[137] Substituting patient-autonomy for physician-beneficence as the basis for medical ethics reduces the need for physicians to live up to a beneficent image. Replacing physician-beneficence with patient-autonomy as a physician's first concern tends to dilute a physician's empathy with patients and their families. Comforting of patients and their families used to be an important function for doctoring, and created the respect and regard for them that is so important for the foundation of the doctor-patient relationship. When patient-autonomy is the goal, doctors will talk to their patients with unalleviated frankness, and act with a lessened sense of commitment. Consequently they become less available, infuriating patients used to physicians' devotion in the past. Patients' respect for doctors weakens and they are less willing to accept their decisions. And physicians are thus less able to implement implicit rationing.

Another side-effect of demands for unconditional recognition of patient-autonomy is that research in treating such emergency conditions as acute strokes, cardiac arrest, and traumatic injuries has been brought to a virtual halt because of the impossibility of getting informed consent from patients with such problems[138].

But, if the costs of medical care are to be controlled, expensive innovations need to be rationed. The question is, how? Blank[6] has devoted an entire book to the theme that rationing of innovations in medical care is a necessity for the economic health of a nation and notes the obstacles that the public places before such a goal. However, Blank[6] and most other observers[131] believe that the economic imperatives involved will make the public reach a consensus on what priority should be placed on health care compared with other expenditures, and on how resources are to be allocated among the various kinds of medical care. Yet, others believe that rationing of innovations, particularly in a democracy, must always be implicit, since "... once a technique is viewed by the public as effective, it's politically impossible to withhold it from anyone."[139]

Finally, the autonomy of doctors in their practice, which has been so useful in implicit rationing to save costs, seems unlikely to survive under the conditions of managed-care and managed competition. Those concepts, which are discussed below, appear to likely to become dominant in the medical-care delivery systems of many of the advanced nations. Managed care and managed competition are thought to promise containing costs and preserving physician autonomy too, but the latter is already proving to be illusory.

B.   Specific Methods for Rationing

Global budgeting is a macro-rationing procedure whose proponents claim contains costs only by eliminating unnecessary care. However, after provider profits have been squeezed to the limit and over-utilization and administrative inefficiencies eliminated, micro-rationing of expensive necessary care is still almost certain to follow. Necessary care needs to be micro-rationed under global budgeting to effectively control expenditures because the single most important cause of accelerating medical-care costs is the increased care generated by innovations and aging of the population.

Ultimately, when global budgeting reduces the resources available to a provider, the provider must decide who receives care. For instance, one Australian hospital, trying to stay within its budget, had to decide which life-saving drugs it could afford, determining that those which cure rare diseases affecting only a very few patients needed to be eliminated[102]. Thus, rationing (or, euphemistically, either the allocation of medical-care resources or priority-setting) brings into sharp focus the conflict between practitioners' responsibilities to the individual and to the society in which they live.

Still another example of an adverse micro-rationing practice resulting from global budgeting of hospitals is that they tend to retain less sick patients longer than necessary to avoid admitting more costly sicker patients who, as a result, are forced to queue even longer[45].

Single-payer plans, of which the Canadian and English medical-care delivery systems are the best examples, also function wherever insurance payers backed by government can negotiate with providers in concert, as in most other advanced countries except, most prominently, the U.S. Single-payer systems macro-ration by setting global budgets for medical care. They also improve the ability to negotiate with providers, because single-payer plans eliminate the possibility of providers playing one source of their payments against another. In some nations the government provides all funds or insurance for the vast majority of their populations, virtually eliminating private insurance companies and markedly reducing costs of administering the delivery of medical care.

Deterrence mechanisms are ubiquitous cost-containment measures that implicitly micro-ration medical care as by limiting the amount of facilities (requiring patients to queue for services) and regionalization of facilities (distancing them from much of the population). Deterrent mechanisms are purported to eliminate only unnecessary care, but, as will be shown they, too, most often also reduce the use of necessary care. That rationing-by-deterrence can act as a constraint on consumption so that "a patient does not receive all the care that ... would be of benefit" was noted over a decade ago[2].

If in fact all rationing-by-deterrence deprives anyone of necessary care, acceptance of their legitimacy then, in great measure, depends on one's attitude as to what constitutes "cost-effectiveness studies" of medical-care procedures. This has been discussed more fully above, on page 32, especially as to what constitutes "futile treatment" and that an expense-to-patient ratio may not be sufficiently cost-effective to justify development of a new treatment, such as gene-therapy.

Since rationing-by-deterrence methods do not restrict necessary care openly (or it's even denied by its proponents that they ever do), their function to reduce necessary care is not "visible" to the public and they should be classified as implicit micro-rationing. The delivery of medical care as determined by the ability of the individual to pay for it (*marketplace rationing*) has always been deplored because it contains costs by deterrence in the use of necessary care. Rationing-by-the-marketplace is of the implicit variety because it is not implemented by legislation or governmental regulation. Medical care in the U.S. continues to be rationed in great measure by the marketplace despite the many efforts to circumvent it. Denial of insurance benefits to those not covered by an employer and not sufficiently affluent to pay premiums for insurance out-of-pocket is a form of deterrent rationing by the marketplace that deprives 38 million people of access to medical care.

Other deterrent methods recognized as containing costs by reducing necessary care as well as unnecessary care are copayments or deductibles required before insurance take over in payment for services, delays in scheduling appointments or admission to the hospital (queuing), and limiting what tests can be done or when they can be done.

Copayments **and** *deductibles* are used to give incentive to the individual to reduce utilization of medical services. They do not deter the more affluent from obtaining services, but they do inhibit the less affluent, often from seeking even necessary care. When they reduce the use of necessary care, copayments and deductibles are then rationing-by-deterrence mechanisms and a form of micro-rationing by the marketplace. A recent example of this entire process is Germany's 1993 medical-care reform act which increased prescription drug copayments in an effort to keep expenditures on drugs within their budgeted amounts[140].

Queuing, another example of "rationing-by-deterrence or delay"[141], is a more obvious, but still an implicit form of micro-rationing and is most notable where the single payer system is in effect, as in Great Britain and Canada. It acts to carry out the macro-rationing decision of government expressed in its global budget for medical care. Queuing means that patients are forced to wait for prescribed, usually non-emergency, treatments. Very often patients for one reason or another are not treated, or have to wait an inordinate length of time for treatments to improve their quality-of-life. Queuing especially holds in check expenditures for new technologies. In Britain, where the NHS provides superb primary care, global budgeting limits specialty care for which patients must queue a long time[142]. Thus for example, since the number of oncologists is limited, Britain's statistics for survival from cancer are poorer than those of other O.E.C.D. nations[141]. The number of coronary by-passes, hip-replacements, dialysis treatments, etc. are likewise limited in Great Britain, and in Canada too, as compared with the U.S.[143].

While additional, and probably affordable, expenditure might relieve queuing, democratic governments usually are loath to increase taxes for that purpose. The affluent manage to avoid the queue by paying for private medical care out-of-pocket, either directly or most often through private insurance. Despite the patent inequality that results, many policy experts believe this turning to private care is desirable, because it both shortens queues and removes from the system those most apt to complain[144].

Cost-containment measures less readily identified as also hindering necessary care by deterrence are regionalization of facilities, the more recently introduced "managed care", and restrictions on the number of physicians produced.

Regionalization is, and long has been, recommended by policy experts as a means of containing costs[45,142]. It has been advanced the farthest in countries where government have the greatest control of the medical-care delivery system, as in Great Britain and Canada. Regionalization has been least utilized in the U.S., and what efforts in this direction have been made, have been through *Certificate-of-Need (CON)* programs.

CON programs were designed to control capital expansion of hospitals. They require governmental agency approval for sizable capital expenditures, and issuance of a CON before adding to or altering a hospital, or before acquiring proposed equipment. States administer the program according to guidelines issued by the U.S. Department of Health and Human Services. The guidelines are meant to prevent costly excess capacity and duplication of services.

Originally, under the program, a hospital wishing to make a capital expenditure of more than $100,000 had to obtain a CON. In 1985 the threshold was raised to $275,000 for any new equipment, $400,000 for any medical technology system, and $680,000 for renovations. Federally-funded local committees of state health systems agencies decide whether to grant the CON, and the decisions are then reviewed by the state Secretary of Health. However, over the years, this program has had little effect on curtailing hospitals' investments in new facilities because hospitals, with local political pressures, often succeed in circumventing the CON purpose.

The dissemination of expensive medical-care innovations resulting from the American free-enterprise system is constantly decried as wasteful. This practice is condemned because it has led to facilities being under-utilized, and used unnecessarily to maximize profits for their investors or even just to cover their costs. Denounced in particular is the conflict of interest that is created when doctors invest in technology and then refer their patients to it (self-referrals). The U.S. Congress has acted against this latter practice but, as of 1995, the Health Care Financing Administration had not yet issued regulations to implement this legislation.

A supporting claim for regionalization is that, concentration of activity, especially in the matter of surgery, leads to greater expertise and better results[145,146]. Regionalization, therefore, improves the quality of medical care. These studies revealed that surgeon volume is far more important than hospital volume. However, the data also suggests that there is no improvement in results beyond a certain minimum level of a surgeon's activity as exemplified by observations on cardiac by-pass surgery. Apparently the mortality-rates are no worse when only one cardiac bypass operation per week (50 per year) is done by surgeons than when surgeons do three, or more, per week (150 or more per year). That minimum level of activity is achieved by many more facilities and surgeons (certainly making medical care much more accessible) than most regionalizers would recommend. Studies on other types of procedures confirm that good surgeons can obtain good results with relatively few patients per year "whereas not so good surgeons may continue to produce worse results however many operations they do."[147]

Most importantly, a recent examination of all reports over the years on the relationship between volume of coronary artery bypass graft surgery and hospital death rates concluded that: "the more differences in case mix are taken into account, the smaller are the apparent benefits of increased volume of surgery"; and, therefore, "policy makers should not assume", as many do, "that concentrating surgical services into larger and more active units will improve outcomes."[148]

It is argued that, if the costs of medical care are to be controlled, expensive innovations need to be rationed in other ways, since most agree that even regionalization would not be sufficient. The journal *Health Affairs* devoted its 1994 summer issue to the problem posed by the insatiable demand for medical innovations, despite their great expense. Direct efforts to regulate the supply of medical technology to the marketplace have been largely discredited: "The required regulatory apparatus is substantial, the political distortions of decision making are likely to be great, and the probable outcomes are ineffective at worst and uneven at best."[149] But Rettig[149] believes, in order to contain costs, the rate of introduction of medical innovations should be slowed. He recommends more careful monitoring of the product development strategies of the pharmaceutical, biotechnology, and medical device industries and in tightening the boundary between new and existing technology. Constraining investment in medical research and strengthening technology assessment would also help. Aren't these really new rationing-by-deterrence suggestions?

Since generalists use far less technology than specialists, others suggest, to slow the use of innovations, increasing the number of primary physicians in proportion to specialists[45]. The tacit assumption is that the effect on the quality of care would not be harmful. However, according to Nelson[46], that is most certainly not true.

Sisk and Glied[45] also believe that fewer, more regionalized hospitals would lessen the use of new technology. While easy access to profitable technology no doubt leads to overuse, it is not often recognized that regionalization can be a rationing-by-deterrence mechanism with harmful effects to some individuals. What is generally unrecognized is that all regionalization, admittedly a useful technique to hold down costs, may also interfere with access to necessary medical care, and thus reduce the quality of medical care. All practicing physicians know that easy access to facilities shortens the time for making a diagnosis and reduces delay in treatment, factors that diminish lengths of disability and suffering. Distancing facilities from much of the population by regionalization will deter the use of innovative facilities even for necessary care.

For instance, people with heart attacks taken to hospitals without cardiac catheterization or cardiac surgery have the use of these innovations far less often than do similar patients in hospitals with such facilities[150,151]. Furthermore, the use of these innovations is inversely related to the distance between the initial hospital without such facilities and the nearest hospital where they are available. In other words, the shorter the distance between a cardiac patient and a catheterization laboratory, or where cardiac surgery is performed, the more likely these innovations will be utilized for them. The importance of easy access to these innovations for treatment of heart disease is emphasized by recent reports that these new treatments for acute myocardial infarction often need to be done within four hours of the onset of symptoms[152].

Incidentally, it also has been reported that coronary revascularization was done twice as frequently for patients with private fee-for-service insurance than for patients under managed care[153]. While there is little doubt that in a fee-for-service environment innovative technology is overused, nonetheless there is considerable positive sentiment reported for the use of coronary visualization and recanalization after acute myocardial infarction[151,152,154]. While the magnitude is not known, it seems clear that there are early survival benefits from invasive procedures in the treatment of acute myocardial infarction[155]. These observers noted several important items to be determined: whether this more aggressive revascularization therapy is justified in light of a higher complication rate, and the additional cost; and determining precisely what are the long-term effects, since the beneficial impact of revascularization may be observed only after 6 to 18 months.

The same inverse relationships between the frequency with which patients received computerized axial tomographic (CAT) scans and the distance of machines from them were disclosed in a study done in California[156]. The availability of an imaging technique on the premises of a hospital to which stroke patients are admitted is crucial, for instance, in differentiating between intracranial hemorrhage and infarction for proper use of anti-coagulants in their treatment[157]. The point is that this differential diagnosis can be made clinically in only a minority of patients and, without an imaging scan, a doctor can never be certain of the cause of a stroke.

Efforts to regionalization are enthusiastically supported by established medical centers, especially of the academic variety. The medical centers base their support on their expertise, derived from their teaching and research, that will assure the quality of medical care. Their prestige and, in the U.S., their deep-pockets[158] give great weight to their support. Empirical studies, on the presumption of better results from greater expertise in academic medical centers, are now being done. So far, reports from New York and Pennsylvania on statewide results of coronary-by-pass surgery tend to dispute the claims that medical centers do better than most regional tertiary facilities. (Perhaps, the training obligation of academic medical centers obscures the presumed greater skill of their faculty[159,160]?)

In the U.S., the academic medical centers were firm supporters of the CON program. This often provoked a catch-22 situation which frequently limited dissemination of innovations. By their very mission, academic centers established experience with innovations before they could possibly be disseminated to district centers and then, when outlying hospitals applied for a CON for an innovation, one important criterion would be that the outlying hospital had had a high level of experience with the innovation.

A fundamental motive of the academic medical centers in favor of regionalization is also to maintain their economic base[158], and possibly gain even greater hegemony in their service area, as has become most evident from their bitter competition with each other in recent years, particularly in eastern cities of the U.S. where they had become bunched together a century ago.

The evolution in the teaching and delivery of medical care over the last 150 years has unintentionally functioned as an implicit rationing method by causing dislocations in the supply of advanced levels of medical care and depriving some patients of such advanced care simply by making access to it inconvenient. The clumping of teaching hospitals bunched tertiary care in large cities, but lessened inner city inhabitants' access to primary care[161]. This dislocation of care is called "adverse rationing" because non-urban populations have less access to tertiary care, while the inner city population has less access to primary care. The problem hasn't yet been directly considered in the U.S. England, which has addressed itself to it, is having difficulty implementing changes recommended by its Tomlinson Report for the city of London, even though full implementation of the report would repair only part of the problem[162].

When medical schools were first established in the 18th and 19th Centuries, people were not treated in hospitals and, as a consequence, hospitals played no role in medical school curricula[163]. Moreover, it was not until after World War II that the innovative revolution really took off in therapeutic medicine. Before then, therapeutic care had relatively little impact. Therefore at the time, the concentration of medical schools in the inner cities had no direct effect on the availability of medical care facilities to people in suburban and more remote areas.

By the end of the 19th century, clinical medical teaching began to take place in hospitals. Medical school teaching hospitals, where tertiary resources became most heavily concentrated, also were gathered in the inner cities. At the same time, inner cities lost their general practitioners and inner city residents had less access to primary care. Such "adverse rationing" also, early on, deprived people in smaller cities and rural areas of ready access to new technology, thus the location of teaching hospitals, inadvertently, became a rationing-by-deterrence mechanism for much of tertiary care.

The free enterprise system in the U.S., together with its local political clout, has repaired this "adverse rationing" with regional hospitals developing tertiary facilities. Much effort is now being expended by academic medical centers, aided by their prestige and financial resources, to counter this deployment of tertiary facilities[158]. The academic medical centers are wooing practitioners to join networks in their employ, and they are merging with, and buying, smaller hospitals. It is not clear how this will work out, since it may be anticipated outlying hospitals with tertiary capabilities will resist being weakened or reduced to only secondary care facilities. Moreover, it is not now clear what role the managed-care entities such as HMOs, which are constantly strengthening, will play in the struggle of the academic centers to maintain and strengthen their role in supplying tertiary medical care.

To repeat, where regionalization has been carried out most extensively, as in England and Canada where governments most comprehensively control the delivery of medical care, queuing has resulted and the public receives much less tertiary care. In their haste to assign the motive of greed to any free-enterprise endeavor that opposes de-regionalization, many policy makers overlook the often beneficial result of the free-enterprise system that results from the marketplace setting the amount of facilities, and bringing them closer to patients. As a result, there is no queuing and the quality-of-care improves for the majority of, even if not for all, the people (as in the U.S.).

It is argued that regionalization is more just because the resources it conserves can be used to make some of medical care affordable to an entire population. This reasoning had evoked support for regionalization from most progressive-minded people - due, in part, to their tacit understanding that a cooperative social project ought to be more fair than any competitive capitalist endeavor. Such an argument can be countered with the suggestion that efforts, used to deprive some of excellent care so that all can have some care, would be better used making the workings of the free-enterprise system give excellent care to everyone. Indeed, recent history would suggest this latter recommendation is more likely to succeed than relying on an ideal that has proven to be impractical: it now has been proven that, so far, the free-enterprise capitalist economy has been better able to increase a nation's standard-of-living than a centrally-planned socialist system. It is possible, then, that this recent historical lesson will erode much of the support for regionalization that had rested until recently on the presumption that the greater justice of planned distribution can provide a better standard of medical care, on the average, for everyone. While a 100% of Canadians and the British, since everyone is insured, have greater access to medical care than do 20% of Americans who are poor, nevertheless, because of the *laissez-faire* growth and distribution of American medical-care facilities, 80% of U.S. citizens have more convenient and more prompt access to medical care than 90% of British and Canadians.

Recently, in the U.S., efforts of insurers (including government programs) to contain costs through managed care (see page 60) has led hospitals to merge. The hospitals justify their merger proposals on the basis of the advantages of regionalization.

Mergers often have been opposed by the Federal Trade Commission, and other governmental anti-trust enforcement agencies, on the grounds that it stifled competition. When blocking proposed mergers, the enforcement agencies have ruled that the resulting loss of competition, in the long run, would leave communities vulnerable to increased costs and lower quality. This would be especially true in markets where only one or two hospitals remained. Hospital representatives have argued the reverse: mergers are of greater advantage to a community than any longer term threat to competition. It is not clear, when evaluating the effect of any particular hospital merger on quality of care, whether the downside effects of regionalization's rationing-by-deterrence factors care are considered. It is probable that the only consideration in these mergers is the cost savings accomplished and the proven economic dictum -- where monopoly exists, the stimulus to compete by improving the quality of the product is lacking -- is overlooked, or is denied.

Pre-, or prospective, payment, methods for the remuneration of providers, instead of the fee-for-service method, are likely to lead to deterrence to the providers in their supplying of medical care. Prepayments, payments made prospectively for services, have been introduced to counteract the excesses in utilization of services previously provided insured patients. Medical insurance which pays fees retrospectively for individual services created an incentive to maximize services. So far, pre-payment mechanisms have been introduced by Medicare for hospital care (prospective payments based on "diagnostic related group" data, or DRGs), and for total care ("managed care") by a variety of insurers, which comprehends medical as well as hospital care.

Prospective payments gives incentive to providers to minimize services they purchase for patients, because giving less service   maximizes the portion of the payments providers can retain as profit. In the instance of hospitals reimbursed prospectively on the basis of the patient's diagnosis, the shorter the stay (also permitting the greater turnover per bed) and the fewer the services provided below the average for a hospitalized patient with a specific diagnosis, the greater are hospital profits. On the other hand, the longer the stay or the more services provided the patient over the average for the diagnosis in question, the greater would be the hospital's loss. Managed care is when an insurance company (health management organization, or HMO) is paid prospectively a *per capita* premium for a patient's total care. Under managed care, insurance company managers and physicians alike are motivated to be as parsimonious as possible in the delivery of care so as to maximize their portion of the capitated "up front" premium payments that finance their enterprise. The incentive of "the less done the more the profit" is the reverse of the fee-for-service incentive: "the more done the more the profit."

The *Prospective Payment System (PPS) According to Diagnostic Related Groups (DRGs)* was introduced into the U.S. for Medicare from 1983 to 1986. It was aimed to control Medicare's hospital costs, which had grown from $3 billion per year in 1967 to $33 billion in 1982 and, together with Medicaid represented about 45% of an average hospital's revenue. Medicare, like Blue Cross and other insurance companies, had previously reimbursed hospitals for "reasonable costs" incurred in caring for a patient, on a fee-for-service basis, with no set limits. Congress mandated the DRG system when it became obvious that neither hospitals nor doctors would contain costs voluntarily.

The DRG system now classifies patients into at least 494 groups. Groups are determined according to diagnosis on admission to the hospital; age and sex; whether the treatment is medical or surgical; whether there are secondary diagnoses; and discharge destination. Then the hospital's reimbursement rate is determined by a complex methodology which includes factors such as hospital location (urban or rural); local wage rates (since labor represents 70% of hospital costs); and a "case mix index" - which essentially classifies a hospital as community, acute-care, tertiary referral, or related to a medical school or medical center. The latter hospitals also continue under the DRG system to receive extra remuneration from Medicare for their teaching of medical students. The remuneration rate is also affected by the region of the country in which the hospital is located. Two types of atypical patients are allowed additional payments: "day outliers" who stay in hospitals extremely long lengths of time; and "cost outliers" who involve extraordinary costs. Although they bring in extra payments, outliers represent a great loss to a hospital. Hospital outpatient services, certain types of hospitals, and certain distinct units within hospitals (psychiatric, long-term care, pediatrics and rehabilitation) were exempted from the Medicare DRG prospective payment system.

The essence of the DRG prospective payment system is that hospitals receive a flat fee for a diagnostic category no matter what the cost to the hospital. Thus, the shorter the stay and the fewer the diagnostic tests and other services a patient receives, the more the hospital will profit from the admission. Since private insurers usually follow federal program reimbursement patterns, many also adopted the DRG program.

The immediate impact of the DRG prospective payment system was that hospital administrations encouraged and pressured their doctors to reduce the number of laboratory and diagnostic tests ordered on patients, and to reduce patients' stay in the hospital. These pressures aren't detrimental to most patients, but they can be harmful to patients sicker than the average of their DRG. The system, for instance, encourages early discharge of patients, often in unstable condition[164], placing severe burdens on their families. Of course, fee-for-services paid retrospectively to hospitals did lead to much unnecessary over-utilization and markedly inflated medical-care costs. There is evidence - retrenchment of services and increased readmission rates - that the DRG system impairs the quality of hospital care[165].

Early in 1995 the Health Care Financing Agency (HCFA) proposed to the American Congress that it extend the PPS to include hospitals' outpatient services to Medicare patients. The HCFA suggested that hospitals' outpatient surgical, radiological and diagnostic services be the first to have their reimbursement method changed, because they represent about one-half of total outpatient charges billed to the Medicare program. The physician payments for these services would not be affected; only the hospital payment would be changed. Up until the time that Congress should act on this report Medicare would continue their payments for outpatient services on a cost-plus basis.

Managed care is a recent effort to control medical-care costs in the U.S. and, even more recently, in other advanced nations - including England and Sweden. Managed care, through prospective *per capita* payments for total medical care, gives incentive to providers to eliminate unnecessary care, but those incentives all too easily spill over to reduce necessary care so as to maximize insurance companies and providers' profits. Some twenty years ago managed care was introduced in the U.S., and by 1994 had grown to involve more than 50 million people, with its greatest expansion in the most recent years and forecasted to continue almost exponentially. Medical care is managed, in the U.S., most typically through health maintenance organizations (HMOs) and similar organizations.

If HMO care does in fact extend its function to limit access to necessary diagnostic modalities and treatments, then managed care, constitutes another deterrent implicit rationing system. The current practice of most American insurance companies still operating on a fee-for-service basis of insisting on prior approval for diagnostic tests and treatments, and most often limiting necessary care, even if only by delay, also constitutes a form of managed care which rations medical care.

Franks, Nutting and Clancy proposed establishing *practice guidelines for physicians* in order to prevent managed-care organizations from underserving their patients[166]. A large industry is said to be forming to develop these standards[167]. It is doubted, however, that enforcing such standards is feasible or desirable; and if they are enforced, it's doubtful they would be effective[168]. In the first place, any such standards should be based on research studies of outcomes and appropriateness of care, which at present are extremely limited[169]. Secondly, the few appropriateness-and-outcomes studies which do exist, have very serious short-comings[170]. Finally, patients and their ailments are so varied that many qualified observers believe physicians' personal knowledge and experience are far more reliable than any set of standard guidelines[171]. Nonetheless, in Great Britain some public health and epidemiologic experts believe guidelines for NHS medical practice are the way of future because of: "the emphasis on audit and improving the quality of health care; medical advances and increasingly complex clinical decision making; unexplained variations in clinical practice; heightened public awareness of, and participation in, decision making; and a more explicit debate about the use of limited resources."[172] Undoubtedly, the implications that practice guidelines have for rationing makes them particularly attractive to those whose primary concern is with the planning of medical care.

Competition with other plans to obtain subscribers provides a second incentive for HMOs to ration-by-deterrence. Such competition compels managed-care companies to lower their premiums as much as possible in order to attract subscribers. Since such companies also compete by benefits offered, they try to keep costs down (and premiums lower) by encouraging parsimonious use of benefits when competition prevents reducing the number offered. As a result, some managed-care entities give explicit directives to their physicians to ration various diagnostic and therapeutic modalities. Such directives, in a sense, could be called macro-rationing, but the implementation of such directives by the managing physicians clearly is implicit micro-rationing. In most cases they would "not need to say anything at all. In other cases, the explanation might be, 'Well, for patients like you the appropriate approach is'..."[173].

It is claimed that managed care, by containing costs and thereby making care available to more people, even possibly achieving universal access, improves *overall* quality of care. But its proponents admit that a small percentage of patients would be denied useful care and, if one focuses on those denied useful care, the conclusion would have to be reached that this type of rationing does not improve quality of care[173]. Also, many observers believe that entrusting rationing decisions to lay managers, or even just a utilization clerk in many instances, will prove far less satisfactory than implicit rationing by physicians. Lay managers would base their decisions on economic expediency, or on presumed public opinions.

Annas recently suggested that managed care might solve the insurance companies' questions about responsibility for the costs of preventive medical treatment for healthy people whose genetic make-up predicts future disease[174]. This problem is likely to be an increasing one with the development of genetic research. Annas had no direct solution to this problem, but speculated that managed care will be "... seen as the primary way to slow proliferation of new 'diseases' and new interventions to address them, and thus the cost of care." He believes even this approach will fail, as will all others, "unless we all will come to grips with our fear of death and our desire to avoid it at any cost to our health insurers." Presumably Annas means that people will have to agree to the explicit micro-rationing of medical care in order to keep within nationally set macro-rationing global budgets. On the other hand, better informing the public and encouraging their participation in rationing decisions could well increase demands for specialty care, and resistance to traditional implicit rationing methods that would defeat the cost-containment purpose of any rationing method, and managed care too[114].

By imposing upon doctors the need to implicitly ration by not mentioning or discouraging the use of available diagnostic methods or treatments, managed care places doctors in an ethical dilemma. Today's physicians are expected, first and foremost, to respect their patients' autonomy by obtaining informed consent. But, managed-care plans, to contain costs, often shorten appointment times (a rationing-by-deterrence procedure) making it difficult to obtain informed consent, a circumstance which requires considerable time for full explanation and discussion of the patient's condition and choices for treatment. The need-to-hurry also compromises the doctor's efficiency and it does not permit the doctor to serve the emotional needs of patients.

Managed-care entities such as HMOs, ration medical care in a manner somewhat like nations with single-payer systems: macro-rationing decisions are made by management and implemented by providers who micro-manage individual patients. Plan administrators practice macro-rationing explicitly, firstly, by detailing in the small print of the contract the number and kind of benefits they will offer. Secondly, they give directives or guidelines to their physicians limiting the availability of some diagnostic and therapeutic modalities to some patients.

Managing physicians carry out micro-rationing for individuals implicitly[173].

Limiting the number of doctors is still another deterrent mechanism for controlling medical-care costs. Medical economists say that each doctor accounts for a measurable amount of medical-care expenditures and, therefore, restricting the number of physicians is sure to reduce costs. In fact, the German 1993 medical-care reforms addressed to cost-containment included limiting the number of medical students to be trained[140]. While the observation on the effect on costs of the number of doctors available under a fee-for-service system with an insured population is clear, nevertheless, an element of rationing-by-deterrence is likely to be introduced when the number of physicians is set by fiat. If medical care were a commodity controlled by the marketplace, the number of physicians would be set by the marketplace too, that is, by the demand for their services. When the number is set by fiat, it would be determined, presumably, by the determination of the needs of the population. However, the requirement to contain costs makes it just as likely that the need for doctors would be underestimated, thereby reducing access to medical care. Those who advocate limiting the number of doctors do so even admitting there is little empirical evidence that it does not affect quality, or admitting they are willing to accept that some patients will be less well served[122].

Chapter 4

What Principles Can Be Used to Ration Medical Care ?

When rationing is contemplated by means other than by the marketplace, almost all observers automatically assume that it be carried out according to the universalistic, rule-utilitarian principle[175]. According to this principle, the morality of an action depends on the extent to which it produces the greatest good for the greatest number. Rule-utilitarianism not only considers the consequences of each particular action, but it also considers the consequences of adopting a general rule for actions. Such a rule should be adopted when it is determined that the consequences of all its actions are better than those of any alternative rule. In a sense rule-utilitarianism is deontologic, or Kantian, since it implies one has a *duty* to act in order to produce the greatest happiness, or the optimum welfare, of society.

According to universalistic rule-utilitarianism, rationing of medical care should demand any necessary sacrifice from old people, because young people have a greater life-expectancy, are more productive and are responsible for children[126,176,177]. In the U.S., such an attitude is encouraged by children's advocates who believe the elderly receive too much of the nation's resources, and children not enough. Indeed, if society's only goal is economic efficiency, then it is better to have as few unproductive individuals as possible. Such a view makes the aged all the more vulnerable to rationing. In fact, one prominent medical ethicist[126] has suggested that we should agree upon an age, somewhere between 75 and 80, to serve as a cut-off for all aggressive, life-extending medical treatment, especially the use of any expensive innovative ones.

Using chronological age as the criterion for rationing is just, some believe, because it would apply equally to everyone[106]. The obvious variability in the health status of elderly people, however, causes medical rationing decisions based solely on chronological age to be a questionable, if not an indefensible, practice. Using utilitarian reasoning to discontinue life-prolonging treatment for the aged who are in some way incapacitated but who still enjoy life begs the following question: why not then also discontinue some younger, permanently disabled individuals, especially low-weight premature infants who, should they survive, are most likely to have permanent disabilities? The permanently disabled young who are unable to contribute to society will have even longer periods of poor quality-of-life than aged people. Thus, even by utilitarian reasoning, there is less reason to prolong their lives than those of older disabled people.

When polled, the majority of people, not being themselves elderly, agree that the old should be sacrificed for the young. When medical professionals are polled on the same question, they concur with the majority, but by a far lesser percentage[23,107]. Yet, in practice, and given the opportunity, doctors too are guilty of ageism (discriminating against the aged)[178]. The term "futility" can take on a different connotation for the elderly. For instance, a treatment that has one chance in ten for helping a patient can be thought to be worthwhile in the young but, even though just as effective, viewed as futile in the elderly[121].

Ageism is even more prevalent abroad, where global budgeting restrictions apply, than in the U.S.[179,180] In England, ageism is particularly rampant, though rarely admitted. For instance, many regions in Great Britain quietly restrict admission to their coronary and intensive care units for those over 75[181]. The belief that the aged benefit less from treatment often buttresses such a policy, despite empirical evidence to the contrary[182,183].

The Royal College of Physicians believes: "There is no biological rationale for the separation of old people from the rest of the human race," and that "Policy should be determined by research and not by prejudice."[184] The Royal College of Physicians also says that using life-expectancy as a criterion for access to medical care is a socially dangerous concept, because the lower classes have lower life expectancy than the upper classes. In fact, lower classes consistently get less care than the more affluent. Even the egalitarian British NHS gives less care to blacks, who have a lower life expectancy, than to whites[185]. While the lessened availability of medical care to minority populations may appear to be solely the result of prejudice, in truth a myriad of associated socioeconomic factors makes it likely to be as much, or more, the result of marketplace rationing, at least in the U.S.[186,187]. Such factors include inadequate financial resources, an inadequate supply of local physicians, poorer educational status and patient choice.

Regardless of the utilitarian concept that favors allocating medical care to the young, the U.S. Government in 1965 enacted a medical insurance program for the aged, Medicare. That legislation was even largely supported by the younger portions of the population. This program was part of the effort (along with Medicaid, an entitlement program for the poor) to make medical care more accessible to the more deprived portions of the population. Even the

Medicaid program, the intent of which was to provide medical care for the poor, has been distorted to benefit the aged. 59% of that program's expenditures is used to supply long term care to 27% of its recipients who are aged. It is true that this aspect of Medicaid, long term care for the elderly, favors the middle classes by permitting them to divest themselves at the end of life to become eligible for Medicaid. Indeed, the possibility of a middle-class backlash was complicating the hope of reforming Medicaid to help curtail government expenditures on medical care (by shaving $182 billion from Medicaid projected spending in the four years subsequent to 1995). This originally was thought to be easily accomplished because Medicaid covers mostly poor women and children who don't vote and have little political clout[188].

When Medicare's expenditures had accelerated explosively to $160 billion annually 30 years after its enactment, President Clinton proposed in his medical-care reform plan that Medicare be cut to help pay for universal access - that is care for the younger, uninsured portions of the population. By 1995, almost all politicians believed the growth of Medicare needed to be curtailed as a necessary step to reduce the national deficit.

One difficulty with using utilitarianism as the basis for rationing medical care is that its guiding principle has two parts which, in practice, conflict. Maximizing the greatest happiness for the greatest number translates immediately to gaining the greatest benefit for the most patients. However, to set a priority between two treatments with the same costs, the choice has to be made between one treatment that might offer immense benefit for a limited number of patients or another treatment that offers a limited benefit for a great number of patients. Another way of analyzing a statement that has two parts, such as greatest good for the greatest number, is that each part is determined by many variables that are unlikely to be consistently true or false for both parts together and, probably therefore, the utilitarian principle becomes unwieldy in the numerous instances for which it is offered as the basis for the micro-rationing of medical care[189].

Others, abroad, warn that the utilitarian concept, which states that the needs of the few must give way to that which benefits the majority, can be perverted by using cost-effectiveness studies to discriminate against the minorities of people with rare or exotic diseases. It is pointed out, in support of this warning, that the NHS is eliminating, or threatening to eliminate, small specialist services, even though they are effective, in order to maximize services for the majority[101,190].

Just as problematical is the fact that utilitarian rationing probably entails discrimination against the less affluent, since the wealthier and better informed in all societies have always obtained whatever care they desired. In fact, many policy experts believe that all systems require an "escape hatch" for the wealthy in order to quiet any opposition to the system, as in the U.K. where, despite any limitations that the NHS might impose, 10% of the population "go private" to obtain promptly any desired care by paying for it with extra medical insurance or out-of-pocket. In recognition of this discrepancy, the 1994 report of the British Labor Party's National Commission on Social Justice called for redress of the inequality of medical care among the different British social classes[191]. This report, however, failed to suggest precisely how to eliminate that inequality.

The recent proliferation of medical-care innovations which have a restricted number of beneficiaries, either because of their expense or limited supply, has evoked a special ethical consideration. Some observers propose not extending these recent innovations to those who are ill because of an unhealthy life-style. For instance, they would deny liver transplants to alcoholics dying of cirrhosis, or heart valve replacements for intravenous drug abusers with endocarditis, or coronary bypass surgery to smokers, despite their prognoses after treatment being as good as non-abusers. Others argue that society or heredity prevent such people from leading healthy lives and, that therefore, all should have equal access to medical care[192].

This last fine sentiment, that all should have equal access to medical care, is in conflict with utilitarianism which requires the sacrifice of the few for the greater benefit of the many. Moreover, the use of utilitarianism as the governing principle behind medical-care rationing creates severe conflicts with the ethical training of physicians. The principle of beneficence dictates that every available worthwhile treatment be offered to each patient, regardless of the cost, and despite any epidemiological cost-effectiveness studies. The recent stress on patient-autonomy as the basis for professional ethics only adds to the dilemma of utilitarian rationing for doctors when the patient demands a treatment regardless of expense[193].

Some commentators contend that rationing should work to the advantage of the least well off[194,195]. The work of the 20th century philosopher, John Rawls provides justification for this approach as an alternative to utilitarianism[196]. Rawls believes that individuals have an equal right to freely choose for themselves. He also believes that a reasonable person would choose that deliberate inequalities be considered unjust, unless they worked to the advantage of the least well off. Reasonable persons would make such a choice because at the onset of any situation they never know into which category they would eventually fall, being "behind a veil of ignorance". Reasonable persons, thus, would opt for the strategy that would assure the least well-off doing as well as possible, for fear they would be in that category. Justice on such a basis would require eased aid to those most burdened by illness, suffering or dinate expenses.

Rawls' theory creates a right to medical care especially for the least affluent. Even though most people agree that equity dictates that medical care be equally available to everyone[185], a Rawlsian approach could justify giving the least affluent more access than the more affluent because of the majority's fear, being behind a "veil of ignorance" when having to choose, that they could be in the former category. Rawls takes great pains to argue that his "rational planner" would place high priority on raising the level of the worst-off in society.

Transcendental morality supplies still another possible approach for rationing (or better, not to ration) necessary medical care. Many people regard life as a sacred gift, and believe there can be no grounds to deny anyone life-prolonging care. To fulfill such a dictate, life-extending care would have first call on all of society's resources. This approach confronts utilitarian ethics that might deny costly care to patients whose illnesses result from ignoring medical advice, such as to stop smoking or drinking[197].

All the philosophical approaches so far discussed, one or another of which are supported by most policy experts, rest on deductive reasoning. They reason from an *a priori* principle to the particular. This deductive approach best describes the reasoning of the proponents for the explicit rationing of medical care. Those who question the validity of explicit rationing can base their opposition on the claim that reasoning inductively from the realities of human behavior leads to the principle that explicit rationing, in all probability, can never be deployed successfully in any modern democratic society. That is because explicit rationing is based on the entire public openly accepting the utilitarian principle that individual advantage often needs to be sacrificed for the general welfare.

Such a proposition demands that individual egoistic self-interest be suppressed, despite the fact that biologic evolution has made self-interest a much stronger instinct than altruism. For instance, William Godwin in the late 18th century ruled that "one must unquestionably save first from a burning house a gifted prospective benefactor of mankind (such as Archbishop Fenelon) leaving one's own wife, mother or benefactor to perish in the flames if necessary"[198]. Could such a rational reaction, purportedly for the good of the species, be evolutionarily incorrect because it places too great a burden on individuals? Even if on the spur of a moment altruism could predominate, over any extended period of time the drip-drip of self-serving emotions arising from the evolutionary older parts of the brain will prevail over any rational formulation for altruism. Altruism, to be constantly dominant, requires unremitting conscious attention to suppress the ego instinct; a pragmatist cannot rely on conscious effort to be so unremitting. Modern pragmatists would not be surprised if people evaded, or disregarded, explicit rationing decisions that deprived them of a possible benefit from medical care.

An anti-transcendental (humanistic) approach to life might also support unlimited allocation of resources to medical care, eliminating therefore, any need to ration it. Such an anti-transcendental theory could support the conviction that there is no special purpose for *Homo sapiens* in the universe. According to this view, humans are the result of the chance concurrence on Earth of oxygen, nitrogen and carbon, which are the essentials for life[199] and the subsequent evolutionary process. The concept that life has arisen by chance out of the laws of physics and developed thereafter by almost immeasurable chance occurrences is more and more agreed upon by most biologists, whether of the "ultra-Darwinian" or "naturalist" variety[200]. If all life is a chance occurrence, then one might reason that there is no purpose to life and, since mankind evolved by chance into being so exquisitely sensuous (because of the power of its expanded neocortex), then evolutionary theory might imply that, in addition to continuing and expanding one's genetic progeny, an individual's purpose is the preservation of its own life. If that is true, then the first priority for all human resources should be for their healthy well-being and longevity. Expenditures for that purpose should be unlimited, and the rationing of necessary care never even contemplated. Such a view is an extension of the Greek hedonistic philosophy, which maintained that life's goal should be to achieve as much pleasure and as little pain as possible.

According to this anti-transcendental approach, since there is no metaphysical purpose for life, there is no reason to subject older people to the stress of being medically abandoned, and age should not play a role in rationing. Otherwise, after being lucky enough to be born in both a society and an era that has given them the opportunity to attain old age, older people would have to pay a penalty for their good fortune. Any practicing physician knows that older people value their lives and, often, their spouse's in particular, much higher than most young people and, apparently some ethicists, believe.

Even some modern utilitarians have decided that the best way to maximize happiness is to maximize individual satisfaction by favoring the individual's autonomous preferences. This reasoning provides a basis for the rights of individuals and their autonomy and thus freedom - including also the right, if they so choose, to expend as much of the resources of society on medical care as will further their individual well-beings.

As if to confirm this modern utilitarian approach, some economists have said, or implied, that the purpose of a nation's economic growth and technological advance is the health and well-being of its population[201]. Since medical care can extend life and improve its quality, they continue, there should be no limitations on its use. In other words, necessary care should not be rationed. Calculations of cost-effectiveness of treatments and preventive measures are always in terms of the number of years-of-life added. The use of "years-of-life-added" as a measure of cost-effectiveness is an implicit support for any philosophical approach that exempts from rationing any medical care that prolongs life and its well-being.

If life developed in the universe by chance, its only goal, then, could well be for an individual's own well-being and to live as long as possible. According to this view the purpose of preventive medicine would be to improve the quality-of-life and to extend it. The function of preventive medicine, then, would not be to conserve resources, as so often is contended[202]. Indeed, the expression of a prevented condition's morbidity, pain, inconvenience or suffering is always in terms of a calculated number of years of the benefited individual's healthy life expectancy. With this philosophical approach, health care shouldn't exist to save money, but to preserve health. This philosophy, that the preservation of life itself is the only purpose of life, provides a reason to conserve our fast-dwindling sources of energy, to develop new sources, and to prevent over-population. Such a philosophy would give these objectives priority over expenditures on armaments[203], and even on most items of consumption. If everyone agreed to this rationale, expenditures on medical care, rather than other consumer items, could become the predominant force in the economics of any society.

Many economists, however, would disagree with the notion: that medical care should not be rationed because life's primary objective is to stay healthy for as long as possible and medical care aids that objective[201]. They base their disagreement on the writings of Adam Smith which states that there are two kinds of economic activities: those which directly produce wealth and those that make possible the other activities in society and have only a secondary economic impact. Health care, education, etc. are in the latter category and devoting excessive amounts of resources to such secondary activities would deprive primary wealth-producing activities of necessary capital. Indeed, depriving wealth-producing activity of capital by excessive expenditures on health care could even end up reducing resources available for health care. Strengthening this economic contention are the observations that the health of a nation's population has been more determined by its economic prosperity than the amount of medical care available[16,17,18,20,22,23]. This point of view, that the large portion of GNP needed to be allocated to support unlimited medical care for a limited benefit to better health, leads to a conclusion that medical care needs to be rationed. Rationed because the resulting savings would be better assigned to other demands on a nation's GNP and eventually improve the economy so that even the medical-care allocation will be improved.

Certainly, opposed to this economic contention for rationing medical care, transcendental and humanistic perspectives can be used to argue for unrationed medical care. The fact is it cannot not be said conclusively that we *must* ration medical care and there are many reasons to think we will never be able to ration fairly and with good conscience.

We do not know enough to resolve the theoretical controversy over whether any national economy has sufficient resources to allocate enough to "necessary" medical care without rationing. Until now, greater concern for other elements that seem crucial to economic success has led all nations to ration medical care, although by implicit methods[204]. In the past, when therapeutic medical care was ineffective this policy was undoubtedly correct because, even looking at individual health, improvement in the health of any nation paralleled only its economic success. Now, however, with therapeutic medical care truly effective, cultural evolutionary pressures may well lead us to reassign our priorities and ration other consumer items so that we can have as much necessary medical care as possible to add to our longevity and maintenance of quality-of-life.

Even if it would be agreed from a theoretical point of view that medical care should be rationed, there is another reason to doubt the practicability of doing it explicitly. It is that governments could never enforce such legislation, and attempts to micro-ration individuals openly can only be ill-conceived. Evolutionist and historical determinists would likely say that individual distinction has always dominated the social structure of the higher species, especially *Homo sapiens*. Therefore, any theory for equalizing the lot of all individuals by enforced rationing of a limited resource is alien to the dictates of human nature and differing abilities of the individual and, therefore, cannot survive any length of time. A society that acted upon such a theory could survive only if the commodity equalized so improves the competitiveness of that society that it clearly benefits a distinct majority of its individuals.

Attempting to ration medical care equitably among all individuals begs the philosophical question: who deserves care? The liberally-inclined believe the downtrodden are not at fault for their condition, and that the government should help them. Conservatives well might regard the abilities of mankind as unequal, and believe that people underprivileged because of their own characteristics should not receive government support, or that such help would be wasted. Many liberally-minded people believe that nurture determines individual characteristics more than does nature, and that human nature is alterable. Liberal people recommend actions that are more reliant on the altruistic instinct than on the egocentric one. Nevertheless, in the early 1990's under the stress of rising medical-care costs, even the more welfare-oriented countries like Sweden and Holland began to curtail their "liberal" approach - and are making the chronically ill and disabled carry a greater portion of the cost of their own care[205,206,207].

In summary, cultural evolution has dictated that medical care be rationed, and that it be done according to utilitarian principles. Many believe that ideal principles mandate that medical-care rationing be done explicitly, but pragmatic considerations lead to the conclusion that its implementation is likely to prove difficult, if not impossible. The attitude, that medical care requires rationing, is prevalent despite several theoretical concepts that, should they ever capture the minds of the majority of people, could dictate that necessary medical care should never be denied anyone and, therefore, never be subjected to rationing.

Chapter 5

Final Considerations

It may be that many people would accept the arguments offered in the preceding section that lead to the conclusion that rationing of necessary medical care should never be contemplated and as much of a nation's resources should be spent on it as is required to supply each citizen with any useful amount. Indeed, two common western democratic cultural concepts can be used to challenge any thought to ration medical care by any means other than by the marketplace. The first is the opinion that all individuals have the right to as much of any item they desire and can afford. The second is the assumption that a nation owes its citizens a decent existence, which can be defined to include medical care in unlimited amounts for the preserving of life and maintaining its quality.

Nevertheless, most economists and healthcare policy experts believe (and the public, politicians and governments most obviously accept) that allocation of resources to the medical care industry does not yield wealth in the classical sense of goods produced and, therefore, should be limited in order not to divert resources from industries that do create value or wealth.

In the U.S., the limiting of medical services has taken place principally through the operation of the marketplace.

In countries which provide universal access, rationing has occurred mostly by other means. The recent necessity of reforming delivery systems to contain accelerating medical-care costs has sparked, even in the U.S., increased discussion of other, non-marketplace, rationing methods. These increased discussions of medical-care rationing have as their purpose the off-setting of any need to raise taxes, and in the U.S., the added incentive of paying for universal access proposals.

Until relatively recently, the great affluence of the U.S. permitted huge expenditures on national and individual budgetary items without the nation incurring too much debt. Now that the U.S. is awash in debt however, its attention is focused on governmental costs, especially the costs of medical care. The U.S. has become snarled in a vicious circle of increasing medical care expenditures on expensive innovations, which contribute to increasing the number of older people who, in turn, require more medical care. Medical expenditures, thus, have so increased in an era of difficult government financing that changes, such as managed care and more competition among providers, are now occurring that are designed to eliminate not only unnecessary medical care, but are sure to ration even necessary care. The conventional wisdom in the U.S. now states that the cost of medical care should not be burdensome, either out-of-pocket or in taxes, and that it also should not prevent the government from shrinking the national debt.

It, thus, may be concluded that the amount of resources to be devoted by a nation to medical care depends upon how much is perceived that can be allocated without accumulating untenable debt and yet be sufficient to extend longevity and preserve the quality-of-life. That has to be done despite enormous expenditures on other standard-of-living items to which populations in advanced nations have become accustomed, and upon the consumption of which their economies depend. This dilemma concisely defines the present U.S. crisis in medical care. On the one hand, there is a moral consensus for supplying universal access to adequate medical care. But on the other hand, there is a reluctance to impose extra taxation, nor is it ever considered to curtail other expenditures in favor of medical care. Since poor people do not live as long as the wealthy[208], Leach recently summarized the American situation to be that: the materialism of the consumer-culture is distracting the population from its moral duty to provide medical care to the entire population[209].

Do the amount and availability of medical care have the same effect on all individuals of a society? If so, a nation desiring only equity must decide how much medical care it needs to raise the health of the less affluent to the level of the more affluent. Recent data, however, question the assumption that merely supplying equal access to medical care will improve the higher mortality rate of lower income people[210]. Economic growth, even if accompanied by increasingly equal access to increasing health care, does not necessarily improve everyone's health[211]; among rich nations, while all mortality rates are improved, they are correlated to the overall amount of wealth. Mortality rates in industrialized countries also correspond to the amount of relative deprivation (or relative poverty) of its citizens. Life-expectancy increases fastest in those developed nations where income differences between the rich and the poor have narrowed, as is demonstrated by the high performing far-eastern Asian economies in comparison with western industrialized nations. Although often not yet as rich, the developed east Asian nations already have better life-expectancy than in the West. Reducing excess mortality attributable to relative deprivation depends on reducing social and economic inequalities themselves, not just supplying equity in access to medical care[23,212].

On the other hand, cultural evolutionists[213,214,215] would say that the proportion of a society's resources devoted to medical care should eventually be determined by what serves its best interests. Since it is not clear exactly what serves a population's best interest in terms of its economic success and health, what will be the best percentage allocation of resources cannot now predictable in the longer term. According to cultural evolutionists, economic competition between nations, particularly democratic ones, will likely determine the allocation and best use of their resources to increase the standard-of-living and well-being of their populations.

Perhaps to this latter purpose is the principle of western mores that the more able and more affluent people have a greater obligation to society than do the less able and poorer people. While the altruism in the nature of mankind supports this principle, it is likewise, undoubtedly, a good principle for a capitalist economy, because it promotes consumerism and enlarges markets. Medical-care insurance, and particularly community-rated premiums, transferring assets from the young and healthy to the old and sickly, has public approval because it is part of that principle. Progressive taxes, which transfer wealth from richer to poorer people, are also favored by the majority, as is the transfer from private to public responsibility of all, or some, of the obligation to supply individual medical care.

While modern democracies have found it popular to voice support to transfer resources, including those for medical care[23,101], from the more affluent to the less affluent, taxation for this purpose is, nevertheless, unpopular. Again, the self-interest of most people is apparently stronger than any altruism needed to impose additional taxation or, now, even community-rated premiums in the U.S. (since they raise the cost of premiums for many voters). As a result, especially in the U.S., legislatures have decreed entitlements for the poor, but principally paying for them by government borrowing rather than by taxation. In the U.S., the national debt is now so large that few consider government borrowing economically feasible. Also, universal access to medical care must be financed by taxation, or else any acceleration in costs needs to be offset by rationing. This problem is all the more difficult because of the public's immense hope in the promise of medical research and commitment to innovations in medical care despite their costs[189].

Transferring responsibility for medical care from the individual to the government brings it into the political arena and places it in competition with other items in the national budget. The distastes for added taxation or increasing the national debt makes the need to ration medical care seem all the more imperative. But, rationing is seldom discussed openly. The reason for this bizarre silence is that even the mention of the term "rationing" is politically unattractive. Rationing is an avoided word because medical-care rationing necessarily involves a clash between individual and public interests. All politicians recognize that, while most people want universal access to care, few are willing to deny their self-interest and vote to be taxed to pay for it or to have their care reduced (rationed), the Clinton Administration recognized this reality when it was forced to drop cost-control measures from its health plan in September 1993 after it was merely suggested that they could lead to rationing and queuing.

As mentioned in the introduction, policy experts often use euphemisms for rationing, such as priority-setting or asset-allocations, to avoid the impact of the R-word on the public. Priority-setting and asset-allocations which, like rationing, mean depriving a relatively small number of people of items of care from which they would benefit. Perhaps asset-allocation and priority-setting are acceptable because they denote macro-rationing procedures, and most people don't understand that, sooner or later, such decisions will involve micro-rationing for them personally.

When politicians and healthcare policy experts in the U.S. propose universal access as part of medical-care reform, they mention neither added taxation nor rationing. Some even say universal access can be paid for by merely increasing the efficiency of the system[216,217]. Others say that competition will lower costs so much that paying for the uninsured won't be very expensive. Reforms that increase administrative efficiency or introduce competition among providers can lower costs temporarily, but the acceleration in medical care costs from expanding *necessary* medical care due to aging and ongoing innovations will continue, albeit from a base lowered by increased administrative efficiency and provider competition[64].

Any proposal to explicitly micro-ration medical-care would be politically untenable. Even in Oregon, where preparations for explicit micro-rationing have gone the farthest, the program explicitly rations the care only of poor people on Medicaid. An attempt to introduce explicit micro-rationing by the NHS in England supplies another example of this process occurring as a political aberration. There, the absence of local providers (and their lobbying efforts) was the reason why three local authorities decided not to provide *in vitro* fertilization. By contrast, three other English districts, that do have local providers of *in vitro* fertilization, do pay for it, and two of these areas even plan to put extra money into that service[218]. Then again, another demonstration of the political unpalatability of micro-rationing is that when arguing for cost-effectiveness as a basis for explicit micro-rationing, policy experts offer only positive examples for it, never mentioning examples of treatments too expensive to fund, or at what level of cost per effective treatment, a treatment is worth a government's ng for it[219].

Another example, admittedly somewhat macabre, of the political distaste to legislate explicit directives for medical care is the fact that all legislative bodies, here and abroad, which have debated legalizing assisted suicide for terminal patients failed to do it[220,221,222]. Some legislators said they were not against assisted suicide, but implied that euthanasia well might be acceptable if carried out quietly by physicians -- in other words, implicitly. In fact, the Netherlands tolerates having more than 2000 terminally-ill patients annually "illegally" assisted by physicians to die[223].

People's objection to the explicit rationing of any medical care has the same origin as their ultimate objection to universal access. Acceptance of such rationing decisions would depend upon the altruism of the majority of the public to forego a treatment that might be of benefit to them as individuals, in favor of greater overall benefit to their entire nation. But, politicians can't rely on such altruistic sentiment to inspire the public to vote to support a utilitarian purpose when individuals are confronted by the possibility of being in the deprived minority. For example, when the public is asked for their priorities for the explicit allocation of medical-care resources, minority groups, like the elderly and disabled, generally need protection, from the younger and healthier majority[101]. Pragmatists, reasoning inductively from the realities of human nature, might well conclude that in a democracy only implicit ration should ever be considered for medical care. That micro-rationing of any extent has only ever been implemented implicitly, supports this pragmatic view.

Nonetheless, many authors favor explicit rationing because they reason, deductively from ideal principles, that rationing done openly recognizes the autonomy of individuals, which is part of the rights of all citizens in a democracy. They oppose implicit micro-rationing by physicians because of the implied paternalism which they believe violates patients' autonomy. Indeed, managed care and managed competition, which are being introduced worldwide in order to limit funding, reduce the role of the doctor in rationing even though they seem to require explicit consideration of priorities in medical care[224]. Policy experts are hoping that public debate about consumer preferences will make explicit rationing an acceptable alternative to the long-standing implicit rationing by physicians. In Holland and Great Britain, the public's priorities are being determined for the various forms of care that providers might supply (as they compete for purchasers)[101,125,225]. Since "determining priorities" must mean that suppliers won't provide the lower-ranked services, this process includes rationing -- even if rationing is never mentioned when managed competition is discussed publicly. Managed care and managed competition enhance the role of managers, and thus, inevitably, their role in rationing. However, this change, thus far, appears to have disturbed, for the most part, only physicians.

A failure to understand changing cultural evolutionary pressures leads otherwise clear thinking policy experts, and many others including physicians, to persist in offering programs for universal access in the U.S. that are not politically possible as the end of the 20th century. The conditions that made universal access easily achievable in most advanced democracies without the need for explicit rationing almost a half century ago, do not now exist[226]. When universal access plans were first introduced abroad, the cost of medical care wasn't as exorbitant as it is today. The innovative revolution in medicine -- which has been a prime cause of the acceleration of costs of medical care and contributed to the aging of the population -- was just beginning in advanced nations.

Before the modern therapeutic revolution, it was possible to introduce universal care since it required only modest individual taxes and employer contributions to finance it. Over the next half century, the incremental rise in costs caused by the gradual introduction of innovations and the aging of the population did not require any sudden steep tax increase in any one year in those countries with universal access, even though costs in these countries have accelerated as much as they have in the United States[65]. Despite similar acceleration and despite their universal access, total medical-care costs abroad have remained well below those in the U.S. That is because their universal care systems, including the single-payer arrangements, preserve and encourage implicit rationing mechanisms, systems that are gradually being dissipated in the U.S. with the deterioration of the physician-patient relationship.

But today in 1995, if the U.S. decided to provide medical-care insurance for its 40 million or more uninsured in one drastic change, the increased taxes and insurance costs to individuals and businesses would seem unbearable, even if coverage were phased in over five or six years. That is, it would be unbearably expensive unless such reform included severe curtailment, or rationing, of benefits. Such rationing would pose a difficult political problem in a democracy where the vast majority have become used to immediately available and broad benefits. Furthermore, efforts in the U.S. over the past 50 years to expand access to medical care -- so that more than 80 percent of Americans now are covered -- is a change that has spawned forces which see reform of the current system as threatening. The medical care and insurance industries have grown so large and profitable in the past half-century that both now can exert considerable muscle to oppose reform.

Every proposal for medical-care reform to the 1994 session of Congress avoided mentioning rationing and would have raised taxes and insurance contributions so much that the public would soon have been up in arms. While community-rating of premiums would have made medical insurance portable and available to those with pre-existing conditions, younger and healthier people would have seen their medical insurance premiums rise to pay for older and sicker people. Many of the proposed plans would have curtailed the growth of Medicare funding so as to lessen the amount of needed taxation to support that program. This reduction, leading to a decrease in (or, a rationing of) their benefits, however, would have outraged the elderly, who constitute a potent voting bloc. Even the single-payer plan -- which in the long run is a transfer from private to public outlays and would save money by reducing administrative costs -- in the short run, to get it started, would impose tax-shock on the middle and upper classes.

It shouldn't surprise us that Congress wasn't able to pass a medical-care reform package in 1994. Legislators, unwilling to lose the next election, refused to vote for a plan that would sharply raise taxes or insurance premiums for the majority in their constituencies. They knew that the majority of voters, who are well insured, wanted neither to be rationed, nor have their taxes increased.

Chapter 6

Conclusions

Most people concerned with public policy believe that it is necessary to contain the costs of medical care, and that its rationing is required. They also prefer explicit rationing over implicit methods and assume that the philosophical basis for rationing should be universalistic rule-utilitarianism relying principally on cost-effectiveness studies for prioritizing the various therapeutic modalities.

The general public, if polled, would surely agree. However, with the exception of the necessity to contain the costs of medical care - reactions in private (such as those in the voting booths of a democracy) and under the immediate stress of illness belie much of the public's alleged support for rationing and universalistic rule-utilitarianism that might deprive them, personally, of a useful treatment. In fact, support for explicit rationing and utilitarianism, which requires some to forsake a benefit for the greater benefit of the many, would demand that individuals be motivated primarily by altruism rather than by their perceived immediate self-interest. Inherited human nature, however, dictates the reverse.

In most advanced nations, the proportion of resources devoted to medical care has generally been 10% or less of their GNP's. This proportion has been exceeded in the U.S. for many years and recently risen to 14%, and is threatening to reach 18% by 2000 A.D. The U.S. medical-care delivery system has been declared to be in crisis, and containing its costs is said to be a national necessity. As a matter of fact, all other advanced nations now, too, are experiencing the same need to contain the acceleration in their costs of medical care. Yet, with medical-care information ever more widespread and with people's instinct for self-preservation, just how much overt rationing of medical care, and the resulting deprivation of some of it, would they tolerate to keep down the percentage of GNP devoted to medical care?

In the U.S., although it is publicly agreed that universal access to medical care is desirable, so far it has not been achievable because it would require the sacrifice, by way of increased taxes or insurance premiums, of a majority of voters to benefit the minority who are uninsured[226]. Most political leaders and some medical-care public policy specialists[227] have demonstrated that they understand the dichotomy between the altruistic public stance and the self-serving private behavior of the vast majority of voters in their constituencies.

For the same reason, the dichotomy between public expression of altruism and the realities of human nature, political pragmatism has dictated that while many democratic nations have explicitly macro-rationed medical care through global budgeting and regionalization of facilities, both expedited by various aspects of a single-payer medical-care system, micro-rationing, so far, has been carried out in all nations only implicitly.

Given the contradiction between most people's spoken attitudes toward rationing and their private agenda, no one can say whether the U.S., or any other democratic nation, will ever successfully implement any form of explicit micro-rationing. Explicit rationing does not appear to be practical - it is incredibly difficult to legislate in a democracy, and would in any case be impossible to make work. On the other hand, the previously ubiquitous and effective implicit rationing by doctors is being irretrievably undermined in the U.S. and, at a less rapid pace, in most other advanced nations.

Yet, even should the present trend to managed care and increased competition drive out unnecessary care, it will still eventually require rationing of necessary care, care that prolongs life and adds to well-being, to contain the increasing costs due to continuing innovations and aging of the population. It is likely, then, that marketplace and deterrent practices will have to be relied upon to carry out implicit rationing, even more than they do now.

In that eventuality, that implicit rationing needs to be increased, the probable consequence will be a guarantee to everyone of only a basic amount of care, and it would be labeled universal coverage. That basic amount would be justified by purportedly equitable, epidemiologically determined, cost-effectiveness studies. Epidemiological determined cost-effective study means that some treatments would not be worth their costs to the entire community even though they are very worthwhile for a limited number of people. The affluent, as always, would get any worthwhile care excluded from basic coverage by buying it either through extra and more expensive insurance or out-of-pocket payments, and by better "working the system". Many in the middle class would likely be willing to trade other standard-of-living items for greater amounts of medical care. Poor, less informed and less aggressive people would get less medical care than others. Many forms of deterrence would, in all probability, be increased to implicitly ration even the guaranteed amount of basic care.

Managed care and increased competition do seem certain to dominate the future delivery of medical care, as they already do in some parts of the U.S. and are beginning to do in Britain, Sweden and the Netherlands. Interestingly, despite the diverging evolution of medical-care delivery systems in western nations over the last 50 years, similar need to contain their ever escalating cost of necessary medical care is now causing these different systems to begin to converge.

Finally, as the proportion of the elderly in the electorate increases, old age in advanced democracies should become a weaker criterion for rationing than at present. Moreover, adding this factor of aging of the population to the reality that medical innovations will continue apace, it is possible that there could be a change in the economic view that medical care needs to be rationed rather than other consumer items less identified with health.

REFERENCES

1. The Compact Edition of the Oxford Dictionary. 1971, Oxford University Press, New York.
2. Mulloy AG. The Allocation of resources for medical intensive care. In Report of the President's Commission on Securing Access to Health Care. 1983, Washington, D.C.
3. Benjamin M, Cohen C, Grochowski E. What transplantation can teach us about health care reform. N Engl J Med 1994;330:858-60.
4. Reinhardt UE. Coverage and access to health care reform. N Engl J Med 1994;330:1452-3.
5. Menzel PT. Strong Medicine: The Ethical Rationing of Health Care. 1990, Oxford University Press, New York. p 3.
6. Blank RH. Rationing Medicine. 1988, Columbia University Press, New York, chap 1.
7. Rationing in Action. 1993, BMJ Publishing Group, London.
8. Hunter DJ. Rationing Dilemmas in Healthcare. 1993, National Association of Health Authorities and Trusts, Birmingham.
9. Honingsbaum F, Calltorp J, Ham C, Holmstrom S. 1995, Priority Setting for Healthcare, Radcliffe Medical Press, Oxford.
10. Brook RH. Health, health insurance, and the uninsured. JAMA 1991;265:2998-3002.
11. Reinhardt UE. The future of the medical enterprise: perspectives on resource allocation in socialized markets. J Med Educ 1980;55:311-24.
12. Evans RW. Health care technology and the inevitability of resource allocation and rationing decisions, Part II. JAMA 1983;249:2208-22.
13. Blendon RJ, Donelan K, Hill CA, et al. Paying medical bills in the U.S.: why health insurance is not enough. JAMA 1994;271:949-51.
14. Angell M. The case of Helga Wanglie: a new kind of "right to die" case. N Engl J Med 1991;325:511-12. and Miles SH. Informed demand for "non-beneficial" medical treatment. New Engl J Med 1991;325:512-15.

15. Dasgupta P. An Inquiry into Well-Being and Destitution. 1993, Clarendon Press, Oxford, Oxford University Press, New York. 94;343:221-2.

16. Charlton BG. Is inequality bad for the national health? Lancet 1994;343:221-2.

17. Phillimore P, Beattie A, Townsend P. Widening inequality of health in northern England. BMJ 1994;308:1125-8.

18. Power C. Health and social inequality in Europe. BMJ 1994;308:1153-6.

19. Lahelma E, Arber S. Health inequalities among men and women in contrasting welfare states. Eur J Public Health 1994;4:213-26.

20. Wilkinson RG. Income distribution and life expectancy. BMJ 1992;304:165-8.

21. Eyles J, Birch S. Population needs-based approach to health-care resource allocations and planning in Ontario. A link between policy goals and practice? Can J Pub Health 1993;84:112-7.

22. Townsend P, Davidson N, Whitehead M. The Black report and the health divide. 1982, Harmondsworth: Penguin, London.

23. Smith GD, Egger M. socioeconomic differentials in wealth and health. BMJ 1993;307:1085.

24. Klein R. Dimensions of rationing: who should do what? BMJ 1993;307:309-11.

25. McKeown T. The Modern Rise Of Population. 1976, Academic Press, New York.

26. Smith BLR. American Science Policy Since World War II. 1990; The Brookings Institution, Washington, D.C., pp.22-27: Industrial innovation and development of technology in the Nineteenth Century.

27. Bell D. The Cultural Contradictions of Capitalism. 1976

28. World's No. 1 Employer: study shows economic impact of travel and tourism. Hotels and Motels Management 1993;208:1.

29. Rosenberg N. How the developed nations became rich. Daedalus 1994(fall);123:127-140.

30. Pauly MV. When does curbing health costs really help the economy? Health Affairs 1995 (summer);14:68-82.

31. New York Times for January 10, 1994, p A1.

32. Healthy people 2000: prevention, federal programs and progress, '71-'92. U.S. Department of Health and Human Services, Washington, DC, 1992, p. 13.

33. Bunker JP, Frazier HS, Mosteller F. Improving health: measuring effects of medical care. Milbank Q 1994;72:225-58.

34. Mackenbach JP, Looman CWN, Kunst AE, Habbema JO, van der Maas PJ. Post-1950 mortality trends and medical care: gains

in life expectancy due to declines in mortality from conditions amenable to medical intervention. Soc Sci Med 1988;27:889-94.

35. Syme SL. The social environment and health. Daedalus 1994(fall);123:79-86.

36. Daedalus: Health and Wealth. 1994(fall);Vol.123: No.4

37. Dean M. Beveridge revisited and restructured. Lancet 1994;344:1285.

38. Judge K. Beyond health care: attention should be directed at the social determinants of ill health. BMJ 1994;309:1454-5.

39. Wolfson MC. Toward a system of health statistics. Daedalus 1994(fall);123:181-95.

40. Evans RG. Health care as a threat to health: defense, opulence, and the social environment. Daedalus 1994(fall);123:21-42.

41. Ikegami N. Efficiency and effectiveness in health care. Daedalus 1994(fall);123:113-25.

42. Baumol WJ, Blinder AS. Economics: Principles and Policy. 3rd ed. 1985, Harcourt, Brace, New York. also, Health reform can't cure high costs. N.Y. Times for August 8, 1993, p. F13.

43. Lamm RD. Medical research: alternative views. Science 1993;262:1497.

44. Grumbach K, Bodenheimer T. Painful vs painless cost control. JAMA 1994;272:1458-64.

45. Sisk JE, Glied SA. Innovation under federal health care reform. Health Affairs 1994 (summer);13:82-97.

46. Nelson GD. Preserving the milieu for medical innovation. Health Affairs 1994 (summer);13:112-4.

47. Huntington J, Connell FA. For every dollar spent - the cost-savings argument for prenatal care. N Engl J Med 1994;331:1303-7.

48. Mant D. Prevention. Lancet 1994:344:1343-6.

49. Fries JF, Koop CE, Beadle CE, et al. Reducing health care costs by reducing the need and demand for medical services. N Engl J Med 1993;329:321-5.

50. The Philadelphia Inquirer for September 16, 1993, p A8.

51. Lasker RD, Lee PR. Improving health through health system reform. JAMA 1994;272:1297-8.

52. Russell LB. The role of prevention in health reform. N Engl J Med 1993;329;352-4.

53. McCormack JS, Skrabanek P. Coronary heart disease is not preventable by population interventions. Lancet 1988;ii:839-41.

54. Strandberg TE, Salomaa VV, Naukkarinen VA, Vanhanen HT, Sarno SJ, Miettenin TA. Long-term mortality after 5-year multi-

factorial primary prevention of cardiovascular disease in middle-aged men. JAMA 1991;266:1225-29.

55. McCormack J. Health promotion: the ethical dimension. Lancet 1994;344:390-1.

56. van Rossum E, Frederiks CMA, Phillipsen H, Portengen K, Wiskerke J, Knipschild P. Effects of preventive home visits to elderly people. BMJ 1993;307:27-32.

57. Field K, Thorogood M, Silagy C, Normand C, O'Neill C, Muir J. Strategies for reducing coronary risk factors in primary care: which is most cost effective? BMJ 1995;310:1109-12.

58. Toon PD. Health checks in general practice. BMJ 1995;310:1083-5.

59. Levinsky NG. The organization of medical care: lessons from the Medicare End Stage Renal Disease Program. N Engl J Med 1993;329:1395-9.

60. Fuchs VR. No pain, no gain: perspectives on cost containment. JAMA 1991;269:631-3.

61. Schwartz WB. The inevitable failure of cost-containment strategies: why they can only provide temporary relief. JAMA 1987;257:220-4.

62. Kirschner MW, Marincola E, Teisberg EO. The role of bio-medical research in health care reform. Science 1994;266:49-51.

63. Grumbach K, Bodenheimer T, Himmelstein DU, Woolhandler S. Liberal benefits, conservative spending: the Physicians for a National Health Program Proposal. JAMA 1991;265:2549-54.

64. Shenkin HA. Medical Care Reform: A Guide to Issues and Choices. 1993, Oakvale Press, Santa Monica, CA. p 18.

65. Newhouse JP. Medical care costs: how much welfare loss? J Economic Perspectives 1993;6:3-21.

66. Letsch S. Health spending in 1991. Health Aff 1993 (Spring);12:94-110.

67. Eddy DM. Health system reform: will controlling costs require rationing services? JAMA 1994;272:324-8.

68. Enthoven AC. Reflections on the Management of the National Health Services. 1985, Nuffield Provincial Hospitals Trust, London.

69. Ellwood PM, Enthoven AC, Etheridge L. The Jackson Hole initiatives for a twenty-first century American health care system. J Health Econ 1992;1:149-168.

70. National Economic Research Associates. Financing Health Care with Particular Reference to Medicines. 1993, NERA, London.

71. Klein R. Health care Reform. The Global search for utopia: no single resolution is likely to work everywhere. BMJ 1993;307:752.

72. Judge K, Mays N. Allocating resources for health and social care in England. BMJ 1994;308:1363-6.

73. Raftery J. Capitation funding: population, age, and mortality adjustments for regional and district health authorities in England. BMJ 1993;307:1121-4.

74. Smith P, Sheldon TA, Carr-Hill RA, Martin S, Peacock S, Hardman G. Allocating resources to health authorities: results and policy implications of small area analysis of use of impatient services. BMJ 1994;309:1050-4.

75. Cohen D. Marginal analysis in practice: an alternative to needs assessment for contracting health care. BMJ 1994;309:781-5.

76. Judge K, Mays N. A new approach to weighted capitation: more sensitive indicators of need but important policy questions remain. BMJ 1994;309:1031-2.

77. Health Care Needs Assessment: The Epidemiologically Based Needs Assessment Review. 2 vols. Eds: A. Stevens, J. Raftery. 1994, Radcliffe, Oxford.

78. Field MJ, Grossman J, Lewin M. Issues in designing benefits for health care reform. JAMA 1993;270:1674.

79. Ham C. Health care rationing. BMJ 1995;310:1483-4.

80. Hayward RS, Wilson MC, Tunis SR, Bass EB, Guyatt G. Users' guides to the medical literature: VIII. how to use clinical practice guidelines. A. Are the recommendations valid? JAMA 1995; 274:570-4.

81. Cochran M, Ham C, Heginbotham C, Smith R. Rationing at the cutting edge. BMJ 1991; 303: 1039-42.

82. Pellegrino ED, Thomasma DC. For the Patient's Good: The Restoration of Beneficence in Health Care. 1988, Oxford University Press, New York.

83. Mechanic D. Dilemmas in rationing health care sevices: the case for implicit rationing. BMJ 1995;310:1655-9.

84. Robinson R. Economic evaluation and health care: what does it mean? BMJ 1993;307:670-3.

85. Orchard G. Comparing healthcare outcomes. BMJ 1994;308:1493-6.

86. Delamothe T. Using outcomes research in clinical practice. BMJ 1994;308:1583-4.

87. Robinson R. Economic evaluation and health care: costs and cost-minimization analysis. BMJ 1993;307:726-8.

88.   Robinson R. Economic evaluation and health care: cost-effectiveness analysis. BMJ 1993;307:793-5.

89.   Drummond M. Cost-effectiveness guidelines for reimbursement of pharmaceuticals: is economic evaluation ready for its enhanced status? Health Economics 1992;1:85-92.

90.   Lee TH. Cost-effectiveness of tissue plasminogen activator. N Engl J Med 1995; 332:1443-4.

91.   Szczepura A. Finding a way through the cost and benefit maze: standardized instruments needed. BMJ 1994;309:1314-5.

92.   Rice DP. Cost-of-illness studies: fact or fiction? Lancet 1994;344:1519.

93.   Robinson R. Economic evaluation and health care: cost-utility analysis. BMJ 1993;307:859-62.

94.   Robinson R. Economic evaluation and health care: the policy context. BMJ 1993;307:994-6.

95.   Teeling-Smith G, ed. Measuring Health: a practical approach. 1988, John Wiley, Chichester.

96.   Editorial. Lancet 1995;346:1-2.

97.   Gill TM, Feinstein AR. A critical appraisal of the quality of the quality-of-life measurements. JAMA 1994;272:619-26.

98.   Strosberg MA, Wiener JM, Baker R, Fein IA, eds. Rationing America's Medical Care: the Oregon plan and beyond. 1992, The Brookings Institution, Washington, D.C.

99.   Gillon R. Medical ethics: plus attention to scope. BMJ 1994;309:184-8.

100.   Rationing infertility services. Lancet 1993;342:251-2.

101.   Tymstra T, Andela M. Opinions of Dutch physicians, nurses, and citizens on health care policy, rationing, and technology. JAMA 1993;270:2995-9.

102.   How can hospitals ration drugs? BMJ 1994;308:901-8.

103.   O'Boyle C. Making subjectivity scientific. Lancet 1995;345:602.

104.   Robinson R. Economic evaluation and health care: cost-benefit analysis. BMJ 1993;307:924-6.

105.   Ham C. Priority setting in the NHS: reports from six districts. BMJ 1993;307:435-8.

106.   Garber AM. Can technology assessment control health spending? Health Affairs 1994 (summer);13:115-126.

107.   Bowling A, Jacobson B, Southgate L. Explorations in consultation of the public and health professionals on priority setting in an inner London health District. Soc. Sci. Med. 1993;37:851-7.

108.   Kitzhaber JA. Prioritizing health services in an era of limits: the Oregon experience. BMJ 1993;307:373-7.

109. Pfeffer N, Pollock AM. Public Opinion and the NHS: The unaccountable in pursuit of the uninformed. BMJ 1993;307:750-1.

110. Fuchs VR. The Future of Health Care Policy. 1993, Harvard University Press, Cambridge, Mass.

111. Hopton J, Dlugolecka M. Patients' perceptions of need for primary health care services: useful for priority setting? BMJ 1995;310:1237-40.

112. Birkmeyer JD, Welch HG. Rationing surgery: rules or constraints? Surgery 1993;113:491-7.

113. Grimshaw JM, Russell T. Effect of clinical guidelines on medical practice: a systemic review of rigorous evaluations. Lancet 1993;342:1317-22.

114. Rees J. Where medical science and human behavior meet. BMJ 1995;310:850-3.

115. McCormick MC. Survival of very tiny babies - good news and bad news (Editorial). N Engl J Med 1994;331:802-3.

116. Osborne M, Evans TW. Allocation of resources in intensive care: a transatlantic perspective. Lancet 1994;343:778-80.

117. Menzel PT. Economic competition in health care: a moral assessment. J Med Philos 1987;12:78.

118. Gostin LO. Law and medicine. JAMA 1994;271:1679-80.

119. New York Times for December 30, 1993, P. A1: Jury awards $87 million in a verdict against HMO for denying experimental bone marrow transplant.

120. Woman cites ADA in bid for experimental treatment. American Medical News for August 21, 1995, p 6.

121. Alper A, Lo B. When is CPR futile? JAMA 1995;273:156-7.

122. Grumbach K, Bodenheimer T. Mechanisms for controlling costs. JAMA 1995;273:1223-30.

123. Teno J, Murphy D, Tosteson A, et al. Simulation of potential impact of a futility guideline in seriously ill adults. J Am Geriatr Soc 1994;46:A6. abstract.

124. Emanuel EJ, Emanuel L. The economics of dying: the illusion of cost savings at the end of life. N Engl J Med 1994;330:340-4.

125. Brown SD, Gutierrez G. Lancet 1995;346:456-7.

126. Callahan D. Setting Limits. 1987, Simon & Schuster, New York.

127. Singer PA, Lowry FH. Rationing, patient preferences, and cost of care at the end of life. Arch Int Med 1992;152:478-80.

128. Kramer AM. Health care for elderly persons - myths and realities. N Engl J Med 1995;332:1027-9.

129. Eastman N. Mental health law: civil liberties and the principle of reciprocity. BMJ 1994;308:43-5.

130. Orentlicher D. Rationing and the Americans With Disabilities Act. JAMA 1994;271:308-14.
131. Eddy DM. Principles for making difficult decisions. JAMA 1994;271:1792-8.
132. Bottomley V. Rationing in action. BMJ 1994;308:338.
133. Fisher ES, Welch HG, Wennberg JE. Prioritizing Oregon's Hospital Resources. JAMA 1992; 267: 1925-31.
134. Shenkin HA. Medical Ethics: Evolution, Rights and the Physician. 1991, Kluwer Academic Publishers, Dordrecht, The Netherlands. p 427.
135. Kimball HR, Young PR. A statement on the generalist physician from the American Boards of Family Practice and Internal Medicine. JAMA 1994;271:315-6.
136. Abrahamson S. University student attitudes to a career in medicine. Lancet 1993;342:757-8.
137. Engelhardt HT Jr. A demand to die. Hastings Cent Rep 1975;5(3):10,47.
138. Marwick C. Research in emergency circumstances. JAMA 1995;273:687-8.
139. Reform debate skirts issue of costly new technology. American Medical News for April 25, 1994, p 1.
140. Henke KD, Murray MA, Ade C. Global budgeting in Germany: lessons for the United States. Health Affairs 1994 (fall);13:7-21.
141. New York Times for June 26,1994. p 1.
142. Parker R. Social administration and scarcity. In: Butterworth E, Holman R, eds. Social Welfare in Modern Britain. 1975, Fontana, London. pp 204-12.
143. Schwartz WG, Aaron HJ. Rationing hospital care, lessons from Britain. N Engl J Med 1984;310:52-6.
144. Klein R. Private Practice and Public Policy: Regulating the Frontiers. In: McLachlan G, Maynard L, eds. The Public\Private Mix for Health. 1982, The Nuffield Provincial Hospitals Trust, London. pp. 97-128.
145. Hannan EL, O'Donnell JF, Kilburn H Jr, Bernard HR, Yasici A. Investigation of the relationship between volume and mortality for surgical procedures performed in New York State hospitals. JAMA 1989;262:503-10.
146. Hannan EL, Siu AL, Kumar D, Kilburn, H Jr, Chassin MR. The decline in coronary artery bypass graft surgery mortality in New York State: the role of surgeon volume. JAMA 1995;273:209-13.
147. Editorial: Specialization, centralized treatment, and patient care. Lancet 1995;345:1251-2.

148. Sowden AJ, Deeks JJ, Sheldon TA. Volume and outcome in coronary artery bypass graft surgery: true association or artifact? BMJ 1995;311:151-5.

149. Rettig RA. Medical innovation duels cost containment. Health Affairs 1994(summer);13:7-27.

150. Blustein J. High-Technology Cardiac Procedures: The impact of service availability on service use in New York State. JAMA 1993;270:344-9.

151. Every NR, Larson EB, Litwin PE, et al. The association between on site cardiac catheterization facilities and the use of coronary angiography after acute myocardial infarction. N Engl J Med 1993;329:546-51.

152. Grech ED, Ramsdale DR. Angioplasty and acute myocardial infarction. Lancet 1994;342:191.

153. Langa KM, Sussman EJ. The effect of cost-containment on rates of coronary revascularization in California. N Engl J Med 1993; 329:1784-9.

154. McClellan M, McNeil BJ, Newhouse JP. Does more intensive treatment of acute myocardial infarction in the elderly reduce mortality? JAMA 1994:272:859-66. and Letters-to-the-Editor JAMA 1995;273:1331-3.

155. Van de Werf F, Topol EJ, Lee KL, et al. Variations in patient management and outcomes for acute myocardial infarction in the United States and other countries: results from the GUSTO trial. JAMA 1995;273:1586-91.

156. Morgan BC. Patient access to magnetic resonance imaging centers in Orange County, California. N Engl J Med 1993;328:884-5.

157. Weir CJ, Murray GD, Adams FG et al. Poor accuracy of stroke scoring systems for differential clinical diagnosis of intracranial hemorrhage and infarction. Lancet 1994;344:992-1002.

158. Iglehart JK. Rapid changes for academic medical centers. Second of two parts. N Engl J Med 1995;332:407-11.

159. Petersen LA, Brennan TA, O'Neil AC. Does housestaff discontinuity of care increase the risk of preventable adverse events? Ann Intern Med 1994;121:866-72.

160. Bell BM. Error in medicine. JAMA 1995;274:457.

161. Maxwell R. Other cities, same problem. BMJ 1993;306:199-20.

162. Dean M. Fewer hospitals, bigger medical schools. Lancet 193;341:620-1.

163. Rosenberg CE. The Care of Strangers: The Rise of America's Hospital System. 1987, Basic Books, New York.

164. Rogers WH, Draper D, Kahn KL, et al. Quality of care before and after implementation of the DRG-based prospective payment system. JAMA 1990;264:1989-94.

165. Gay EG, Kronenfeld JJ. Regulation retrenchment - the DRG experience: problems from changing reimbursement practice. Soc Sci Med 1990;31:1103-18.

166. Franks P, Nutting PA, Clancy CM. Health care reform, primary care, and the need for research. JAMA 1993;270:1449-53.

167. Kassirer JP. The quality of care and the quality of measuring it. N Engl J Med 1993; 329:1263-5

168. Kassirer JP. The use and abuse of practice profiles. N Engl Med 1994;330;634-5.

169. Anderson C. Measuring what works in health care. Science 1994;263:1080-2.

170. Phelps CE. The methodologic foundations of studies of the appropriateness of medical care. N Engl J Med 1993;329:1241-5.

171. Tannenbaum SJ. What physicians know. N Engl J Med 1993;329:1268-71.

172. Thomson R, Lavender M, Madhok R. How to ensure that guidelines are effective. BMJ 1995;311:237-42.

173. Eddy DM. Rationing resources while improving quality. How to get more for less. JAMA 1994;272:817-24.

174. Annas GJ. When should preventive treatment be paid for by health insurance. N Engl J Med 1994;331:1027-30.

175. Smart JJC. Utilitarianism. The Encyclopedia of Philosophy. Paul Edwards, Editor-in-Chief. 1967; Macmillan Co. & the Free Press, New York. Vol. 8. pp. 206-12.

176. Daniels N. Am I My Parents' Keeper ? An Essay on Justice between the Young and the Old. 1988, Oxford University Press, New York.

177. Veatch RM. Justice and the economies of terminal illness. Hastings Cen Rep 1988;18:34-40.

178. Lubitz J, Beebe J, Baker C. Longevity and medical expenditures. N Engl J Med 1995;332:999-1003.

179. Do doctors short-change old people? Lancet 1993;342:1-2.

180. Brancati FL, Chow JW, Wagener MM, Vacarello SJ, Yu VL. Is pneumonia really the old man's friend? Two-year prognosis after community-acquired pneumonia. Lancet 1993;342:30-3.

181. The Economist for April 23, 1994, pp 16-17.

182. Levensky NG. Age as a criterion for rationing health care. N Engl J Med 1990;322:1813-6.

183. Chelluri L, Pinsky MR, Donahoe MP, Grenvik A. Long-term of critically ill elderly patients requiring intensive care. JAMA 1993;269:3119-23.

184. Ensuring Equity and Quality of Care for Elderly People. 1994, Royal College of Physicians, London.

185. Whitehead M. Who cares about equity in the NHS? BMJ 1994;308:1284-7.

186. Friedman E. Money isn't everything: nonfinancial barriers to access. JAMA 1994;271:1535-8.

187. Gaston RS, Ayres I, Dooley LG, Dietham AG. Racial equality in renal transplantation. JAMA 1993;270:1352-5.

188. Much ado about Medicaid. American Medical News for August 21, 1995, p 3.

189. Cipra B. Pinning down a treacherous border in logical statements. Science 1994;264:1349.

190. Future of small and specialist medical services in Britain. Lancet 1993;342:316.

191. Dillner L. Commission calls for shake up in welfare state. BMJ 1994;309:1105-6.

192. Higgs R. Human frailty should not be penalized. BMJ 1993;306:1049-50.

193. Charlesworth M. Bioethics in a Liberal Society. 1993, Cambridge University Press, New York.

194. Brock D, Daniels N. Ethical foundations of the Clinton Administration's proposed health care system. JAMA 1994;271:1189-96.

195. Consensus statement on the triage of critically ill patients. JAMA 1994;271:1200-3.

196. Rawls J. A Theory of Justice. 1971, Harvard University Press, Cambridge, Mass.

197. Finfer S, Howell S, Miller J, Willett K, Wilson-MacDonald W. Managing patients who refuse blood transfusions: an ethical dilemma. BMJ 1994;308:1423-6.

198. Midgley M. TLS for June 18, 1993, p 3.

199. Gribben J. In The Beginning: After COBE and Before the Big Bang. 1993, Little, Brown & Co., Boston.

200. Eldredge N. Reinventing Darwin: The Great Debate at the High Table of Evolutionary Theory. 1995, John Wiley & Sons, New York.

201. Frank JW, Mustard JF. The determinants of health from a historical perspective. Daedalus 1994(Fall);123(4):1-19.

202. Caskey CT. Presymptomatic diagnosis: a first step toward genetic health care. Science 1993;263:48-9.

203. Smith R, Leaning J. Medicine and global survival. BMJ 1993;307:693-4.

204. Richards T, Smith R. How should European health policy develop? A discussion. BMJ 1994;309:116-21.

205. Ham C. Health care reforms in Sweden. BMJ 1991;303:1283.

206. Swedes in an identity crisis as welfare state shrinks. Philadelphia Inquirer for June 26, 1994. p C1.

207. Sheldon T. Chronically sick penalized in the Netherlands. BMJ 1994;308:1059.

208. Pappas G, Queen S, Hadden W, Fisher G. The increasing disparity in mortality between socioeconomic groups in the United States, 1960 and 1986. N Engl J Med 1993;329:103-9.

209. W. Leach: Land of Desire: Merchants, Money, and the Rise of a New American Culture. Pantheon, 1993.

210. Wilkinson RG. Divided we fall: The poor pay the price of increased social inequality with their health. BMJ 1994:308:1113-4.

211. Editorial: The unequal, the achievable, and the champion. Lancet 1995;345:1061-2.

212. The Economist for June 4, 1994. pp 55-6.

213. Huxley J. Eugenics in evolutionary perspective. Perspectives in Biology and Medicine 1963;6:155-87.

214. Boyd R, Richerson PJ. Culture and the Evolutionary Process. 1985, University of Chicago Press, Chicago.

215. Degler CN. In Search of Human Nature: The Decline and Revival of Darwinism in American Social Thought. 1991, Oxford University Press, New York.

216. Brook RH, Lohr KN. Will we need to ration effective health care? Issues Sci Technol. 1986;3:68-77

217. Woolhander S, Himmelstein DU. The deteriorating administrative efficiency of the U.S. health care system. N Engl J Med 1991;324:1253-8.

218. Redmayne S, Klein R. Rationing in practice: the case of in vitro fertilization. BMJ 1993;306:1521-4.

219. Bottomley V. Priority setting in the NHS. In: Rationing in Action. 1993, BMJ Publishing Group, London. p 30.

220. Mercy for the Dying. New York Times for May 28, 1994. p 18.

221. Their lordships on euthanasia. Lancet 1994;343:430-1.

222. Sheldon T. Dutch argue that mental torment justifies euthanasia. BMJ 1994;308:431-2.

223. van der Wal G, Dillmann RJM. Euthanasia in the Netherlands. BMJ 1994;308:1346-9.

224. Best G, Knowles D, Mathew D. Managing the new NHS: breathing new life into the NHS reforms. BMJ 1994;308:842-5.
225. Donaldson C, Mooney G. Needs assessment, priority setting, and contracts for health care: an economic view. BMJ 1991;303:1529-30.
226. Shenkin HA. Eventual health reform likely. Health Affairs 1995 (Summer);14:324.
227. Mongan JJ. Anatomy and physiology of health reform's failure. Health Affairs 1995 (Spring);14:99-101.

INDEX